MW00529029

CRYSTAL
PRESCRIPTIONS

Volume 7

The A-Z Guide to Creating Crystal
Essences for Abundant Well-Being,
Environmental Healing and Astral-Magic

CRYSTAL
PRESCRIPTIONS

Volume 7

The A-Z Guide to Creating Crystal
Essences for Abundant Well-Being,
Environmental Healing and Astral-Magic

Judy Hall

Author of the best-selling

The Crystal Bible series

With an introduction by David Eastoe,

Founder Petaltone Essences

BOOKS

Winchester, UK
Washington, USA

First published by O-Books, 2019
O-Books is an imprint of John Hunt Publishing Ltd., 3 East St., Alresford,
Hampshire SO24 9EE, UK
office@jhpbooks.net
www.johnhuntpublishing.com
www.o-books.com

For distributor details and how to order please visit the 'Ordering' section on our
website.

Text copyright: Judy Hall 2018

ISBN: 978 1 78904 052 4
978 1 78904 053 1 (ebook)
Library of Congress Control Number: 2018934826

A CIP catalogue record for this book is available from the British Library.

Design: Stuart Davies

UK: Printed and bound by CPI Group (UK) Ltd, Croydon, CR0 4YY
US: Printed and bound by Thomson-Shore, 7300 West Joy Road, Dexter, MI 48130

Disclaimer
The information given in this directory is in no way intended to be a
substitute for treatment by a medical practitioner. Further assistance
should be sought from a suitably qualified crystal healing or
vibrational essence therapy practitioner or, in the case of addictions,
cancer and similar matters from an integrative medical practitioner. In
the context of crystal and essence healing, healing can be defined as
bringing the body, emotions, mind and spirit back into balance. It
does not imply a cure. Certain stones are regarded as crystal
whether or not they exhibit an internal crystal lattice or may be of
organic origin.

We operate a distinctive and ethical publishing philosophy
in all areas of our business, from our global network of
authors to production and worldwide distribution.

Contents

Volumes in this series

Acknowledgements

I would like to thank Ian White for introducing me many years ago now to his, at the time innovative, flower essence-making as, up until then, I'd only encountered the Bach remedies. David Eastoe of *Petaltone Essences* and Jeni Powell of *The Crystal Balance Company* hold a special place in my heart. Don Denis of The Flower Essence Repertoire who gathered under his roof many of the leading flower essence producers, with whom I was able to study, deserves much thanks and gratitude. Also the essence producers who made that journey to Milland. It was a pleasure to learn from you all. Sue and Simon Lilly have always been a great help so my love and gratitude to you. While I was working as a drug and alcohol counsellor for SCAD, *Spiritual Dimensions of Healing Addictions* and *Further Dimensions of Healing Addictions* by astrologer Donna Cunningham and Andrew Ramer were invaluable in supporting clients in their withdrawal from addictive substances. And to all the workshop partici-pants with whom I have created, tested and experienced essences over the past forty-five years, my love and thanks.

Foreword by David Eastoe,
founder Petaltone Essences

In a world of information technology, it is amazing how hard it can be to find good, useable, safe information on the use of energies for healing of any kind. However, there are a few rare beings in amongst all this who shine like a beacon and do actually know what they are talking about and one such rare soul is Judy Hall. Judy was involved in the very early days of my developing Petaltone Essences and played a major role in forming what Petaltones were to become.

In the early 90s I had begun researching using plant and flower essences to effect change both in the energies of my own aura, and to clear out harmful, negative slow frequency vibrations from the buildings that I had to spend time in, and from crystals that I liked to work with. This involved testing new ways of creating and applying essences, and relied on the input and feedback of one or two key people, for which I am seriously grateful! I would arrive at Judy Hall's place with a bunch of things to test, excited that I had discovered something potentially useful, and eager to see what she thought. Her feedback has helped and guided me through this exploration, and her depth of knowledge and perception extends into realms I have only glimpsed. She has also introduced me to the powerful use of essences with crystals/minerals, including using crystal grids for protection and clearing. I now use these all the time, with excellent results.

To this day, I still send Judy my new essences to test!
David Eastoe

Part I

What is a crystal essence?

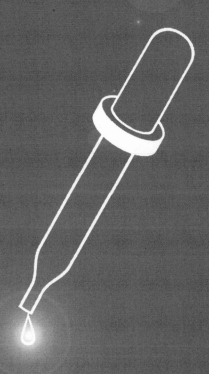

What is a crystal essence?

Essences are essentially nutrients for the soul.
– Mary Wutz

Nutrients for the soul. An excellent way to describe the subtle vibrational healing properties of crystal essences and gem waters. They offer balm and solace to the soul and abundant well-being to the body, psyche and environment. As we will see, they are a form of holistic healing that has been in use since time began and which calls on correspondences established with astrology and astral-magic since its inception.

Modern essences

Crystal essences are an excellent way to use the healing power of crystals, particularly for chakra balancing and higher chakra activation, protection, mental and emotional rebalancing, stress release and space clearing. In this context, it must be remembered that energy healing is defined as 'bringing back into balance' and does not imply a cure. Crystals assist your body, or your psyche and soul, to heal itself. However, essences are versatile and may also assist in manifesting your aspirations and outcomes, supported by the crystals chosen, or take you journeying through the multidimensions of consciousness and the multiverses that surround us. They can also facilitate bringing out the innate potential in your birthchart and assist you to be all that you may be. The possibilities are literally limitless.

At its most basic, a crystal essence is the vibrational frequency given off by a crystal, its 'energy signature', transferred into water. This is achieved either by immersing the crystal in water (the direct method) or by standing the crystal in a container within the water (the indirect method). Or, placed alongside the water if the crystal is large. Essences can also be made by using sound to transfer the vibration to the water – some powerful essences have been made in Tibetan bowls for instance. The water stores the crystal energy-pattern-vibrations and transfers them to the physical or subtle bodies in a similar way to that in which a homoeopathic essence works.

As Simon Lilly explains, "Matter is what our biology experiences as holding patterns, temporarily localised in time and space."[1] 'Dis-ease', in whatever form, arises from an imbalance or disturbance in that holding pattern. An essence restores equilibrium to the core energy pattern. Crystals have a fixed, coherent energy lattice that holds constant. The human body, and the environment, do not. Our vibrations and those that surround us are easily 'thrown out' of balance. By 'entraining' the energies, the coherent lattice of the crystal restores the disturbed energy pattern to equilibrium. As the memory held in the water is short term, it is stabilised by adding a preservative such as brandy. Essences are holistic, that is they treat the whole person *and* the issues that underlie or surround a situation or condition, bringing all levels of being into harmony.

> *Everything on Earth resonates at a vibrational frequency. Frequency basically means the rate at which the molecules, or atoms, of matter rotate around one another, creating an energetic wave or vibration. The human vibrational field operates in harmony with all other beings – animals, plants, minerals and the planet itself – and has to be maintained at a specific level to ensure optimal health and well-being. This synergistic bioenergy, including our auric and physiological structure, can be disturbed by disorganised and disharmonious frequencies. Modern technologies and communication devices rely on electromagnetic waves in order to carry out their function. The frequencies these generate can affect human vibrations, leading to the disturbance of our inner biological clock, compromised immunity and a drop in overall well-being... fortunately crystals return the body to a state of equilibrium.*
> *– Crystal Prescriptions volume 3*

Crystal essences gently facilitate letting go of layers of buried emotions and past-their-sell-by-date thought patterns that no longer serve. These patterns unconsciously create who you are and how you react to situations and people in your life. They can be changed. However, as with a computer, when new programmes are inputted into our energy field through our thoughts, emotions or experiences; when old patterns are overwritten, or the system defragged, remnants of an old programme may remain that distort or clog up the subtle energy field. This may be in the form of a psychosomatic ailment of the body, an imprint or distortion on one of the etheric bodies, or an engram – emotional memory. In other words, a toxic residue can occur on several levels that may require more than one essence to release it. You could look on crystal essences as the means by which your energy bodies are deprogrammed and a totally new operating system inputted as appropriate (see Deprogramming crystal essence page 45 and specific directory entries).

The rare and rather wonderful Rainbow Mayanite is an example of a crystal that repatterns the energy field to its optimum functioning and highest frequency. If even a tiny scrap of toxic or inappropriate energy has been left in the energy bodies, Rainbow Mayanite highlights the last remnant of transmutational work required. Having brought such scraps to your attention, it dissolves them, de-energizes the memory structure left behind, and replaces them with 'divine sparks' of pure energy. As it is a rare crystal, a tiny fragment or the energetic imprint from a high quality photograph (such as the one in *The Crystal Wisdom Healing Oracle, 101 Power Crystals* or on my website) can be used to create an essence that is then added to future repatterning essences without the need for the actual crystal to be present (*see The photographic method, page 61 and see defragging crystals page 44*).

Several, or indeed many, possible crystals are included under each entry in the A-Z directories. This does not mean that you have to use them all. One, two or three crystals up to a maximum of four are generally all that is required. Several crystals may be combined in an essence, provided you choose compatible crystals (dowse to check compatibility, *see page 31*). The synergy can be powerful – if you don't overdo it! Adding regulatory crystals (*see page 52*) assists the essence to work at a rate and vibratory level suitable for the body to which it is being applied. You simply have to ascertain the best crystal(s) from the list for your personal energy field (*see Choosing your crystals, page 20*). If you do find you have a surfeit of crystals that offer to assist, sequential concate-nation could be your answer (*see page 70*) as it strips back layers to reveal the core issue which the final essence resolves.

This book also shows you how to create innovative astrological essences to bring out the potential in your birthchart or facilitate handling challenging aspects and transits – the current movement of the planets overhead. Astral-magic harnesses the power of the celestial spheres to your essences (see pages 145–176).

All the essences within this book are intended for personal consumption (usage). The book is not a guide to creating essences for sale as these must adhere to strict legal requirements regarding production, labelling and the claims made. Such requirements vary from country to country. However, even when creating essences for personal consumption, attention should always be paid to basic hygiene and appropriate storage.

Ancient prescriptions

Drink Bloodstone in wine and poisonous asps defy.
Drink too the changeful Agate in thy wine.
Like different gems its numerous species shine.
– The Lithica

It became clear to me during my Master's degree research a few years ago into the connection between crystals and astrology that crystal healing is not a 'new-age' fad. It's one of the oldest forms of vibrational healing. In Mesopotamia around 1900 BCE, Bloodstone was used for diseases of the blood and was sacred to Mars, as were Chalcedony and Jasper, often used then, as now, for fertility and protection. Selenite, then as now, was sacred to the Moon. Similarly, ancient astrological connections between celestial objects, the hours of the day and night, days of the week and months of the year have carried forward through Arabic and Renaissance magic into the present day. These correspondences still hold good and are the basis for many of the zodiac 'birthstones' and planetary gems.

What did surprise me initially, however, was that, in ancient Egyptian and similar medical texts, instructions were given to gather the morning dew not only from flowers but also from crystals and rocks. Dew from a Malachite left out overnight in the desert was collected to make an eyewash for infected eyes. Malachite having natural antibiotic properties. Similarly, even earlier in the Stone Age, water was collected from pools around the Preseli Bluestones in Wales. The same Bluestones that would later form the sacred heart of Stonehenge. In other words, these ancient people were using crystal essences. Some of the methods continue today, bathing in and drinking the essences, for instance.

A popular method was to pulverise crystals and mix them with liquid to make an elixir for oral consumption. Ancient peoples routinely put crystals into wine, honey (a natural antibiotic) or into oils (many of which had antiviral and antibiotic properties). Pliny the Elder (23–79 AD) called mead *militites* in his *Natural History* (*Naturalis Historia*) and differentiated wine sweetened with honey, 'honey-wine', from mead.[2] All of which are preservatives, of course, although essences were usually created for immediate consumption. The elixirs used were often chosen for their colour – Yellow Beryl for jaundice, red Bloodstone for bleeding and Lapis Lazuli for the blue of restricted circulation for instance. Crystal wine prescriptions were seen by the fourth century Greek Lithica, *Orpheus on Gems*, as being particularly effective against snakebite,

> For wounds inflicted by the reptile race, the Ostrites [Serpentine] mixed with wine affords again a quick relief to cool their fiery pain.

And what man could possibly resist "fresh honours on a

barren scalp", the Lithica's baldness cure using "Stagshorn".° Although, strictly speaking, this appears to have been an organic substance not a stone. The ancients made little distinction between the two:

> *If time hath thinned thy locks, its force shall spread a youthful covering o'er thine aged head. With [Stagshorn] in oil dissolved anoint, and lo! Fresh honours on thy barren scalp shall grow.*

The Lithica also offers a rather poetic way of treating sickly ewes whose milk had dried up – and also new mothers – with milky Snow Quartz. We catch a glimpse of the rituals that accompanied the preparation and use of such stones in those ancient times:

> *When their piteous tale they bleat, bid thy shepherds lave it [Snow Quartz] in the dark pools where sleeps the fountain-wave.*
> *Next, ranged in order 'gainst the rising sun.*
> *With fitting rite thus purify each one.*
> *Take in thine hand a goblet filled with brine. Mixed with this stone reduced to powder fine.*
> *Thy sheep and goats then carefully go through, sprinkling their fleeces with the lustral dew.*
> *Straightway the mothers, of their sickness healed, to their glad young shall milk abundant yield...*
> *And bid the bride, but late a mother made, to drink this gem with honied mead allayed that her sweet infant on her flowing*

breast, drunk with the copious stream, may soundly rest.

Pliny, a first century Roman historian and geographer, whilst tending to disparage crystal pharmacology, tells us a great deal about the use of crystals and organic substances as a healing tool in his and earlier ages. He mentions over two hundred crystals and methods such as "draughts", boiling in wine, combining with honey and even pomegranate juice. The method he describes here uses water as a medium to convey powdered Amber, a natural antibiotic, as an antidote to "attacks of wild distraction" and "strangury" amongst other ailments:

> *Amber is found to have some use in pharmacy… Callistratus says that it is good also for people of any age as a remedy for attacks of wild distraction and for strangury, both taken in liquid… affections of the ears when powdered and mixed with honey and rose oil, as well as weak sight if it is powdered and blended with Attic honey… and affections even of the stomach if it is swallowed in water.*

Equally useful would be the "gold-spangled acopos" if only I could find a modern translation for this crystal name which literally means 'not fatiguing'. The latin-lexicon.org defines it as "perhaps a kind of stone, crystalline quartz or spar" and Jeni Powell's guide Guisseppe suggested Gold Rutilate. Which could be Rutilated Quartz, or the wonderful Hematite and Rutile combination crystal that's been around for a few years.

When heated in oil, so Pliny tells us, it creates "an embro-cation that dispels fatigue".[3] It was prized for relieving stiffness and pain. It sounds like it could also be Magnetite or Magnesite, or possibly a pyrite given the "gold-spangled" element. Not quite such an obscure a name, "ostracites" seemingly translates as fossilised oyster shell. According to Pliny it was taken as a "draught to arrest bleeding", and applied with honey as an ointment to "cure sores and pains in the breast". Boiled in wine, Jet relieved toothache and Hematite created a "universal remedy" and was much associated with blood.[4]

°"Stagshorn" or Hartshorn was not from the antlers. It was believed to be a stone secreted within the brain of the stag.

Using this book

This volume of the *Crystal Prescriptions* series is set out somewhat differently to the usual *Crystal Prescriptions* format in which the A-Z directory is the final section. In this book, to assist you to navigate around the topics, there is an A-Z directory with a selection of potential crystals for particular issues or symptoms following on from the topic heading. So, under 'Addictions' in the Specific crystal essences section, for instance, you'll find not only crystal essences for addictions to specific substances but also for the psychological or physio-logical issues that underlie the addiction. These issues may need addressing, either preceding or during withdrawal from the addictive substance. It is all part of 'peeling back the layers' to reach the core. You will also find remedies for conditions such as codependency and 'poor me' (victim mentality) that so often accompany addiction. In some of the introductory material too, crystal suggestions follow on immediately after a topic as they may relate to more than one section. As always with the directories, choose crystals from the lists that are appropriate to you (see Choosing your crystals pages 20–43).

Why so many crystals?
Literally every body is different and not all crystals will work for you. You need to find a crystal or combination of crystals that resonates with your own subtle energy

field. There is no one-size-fits-all crystal, although Shungite and Brandenberg Amethyst come closest. Therefore, a choice of crystals is given so that you can discover which crystals are uniquely suited to you.

However, do bear in mind that an emphatic 'no' response may mean exactly that, or that there could be an underlying resistance to what the crystal would reveal. There may also be a conflicting agenda between what your physical body and your head thinks is needed and what your soul actually requires. It is possible to work through this by dowsing or intuiting your deepest needs, stripping away the layers in sequence (see page 31), so long as you are aware that conflicts may arise and are prepared to work with these during the ongoing process of healing.

What if an essence doesn't work for me?

It is rare that an essence fails to work but it does occur. Not all crystals work for everyone as we've seen. But most people can find at least one or two that resonate in harmony with their personal energy field and soul needs. It may be a case of applying a little patience and gradually refining your choices. It may also be necessary to discover what lies behind a condition, or an issue that is creating an apparent aversion. There may be deep-seated causes – or hidden blockages. Desperately wanting a crystal essence to work *and/or* being cynical and antagonistic to the very idea are self-defeating. Toxic attitudes and negative expectations may block crystal energies. Disbelief is a powerful block. An open mind is essential. You may need to address the underlying resistance first, opening your mind to possibilities. Or, be prepared to sit back dispassionately and allow crystal energies to work *in their own way and in their own time*. Outcomes may not necessarily be what you thought you wanted. Crystals work for your highest good and that may mean uncovering hidden agendas, ancestral or karmic traumas, repressed memories or emotions and so on. Once these are resolved, you will enjoy much greater well-being. Also, it must be remembered that there are times when your soul has actually chosen a condition or issue through which to learn and grow. In such a case, an essence cannot work against your soul purpose, although it could accelerate the soul-learning process and facilitate evolving and moving on.

If healing does not occur

There are occasions when no matter what type of therapeutic intervention is tried a dis-ease or situation does not improve. This may be because:

- A soul may not have finished evolving through that condition.
- A soul may be trying to 'get better'/find a 'cure' for the wrong reasons.
- A soul may be entrenched in 'reparation-restitution' mode, in other words stuck in 'payback'.
- A soul may have learnt all it needs and leaves so

that it can incarnate again and put lessons into practice.
- A soul may be offering itself or someone else a lesson or an opportunity to change/grow.

However, essences can support the incarnated soul in dealing with a situation with grace and ease, bringing out the positive soul learning rather than setting up negative karma.

Part II
Choosing your crystals

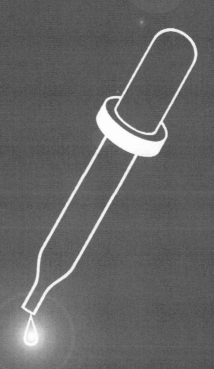

Choosing your crystals

Choosing your crystals is the start of the essence-creating process. There are several methods. Not every crystal suits every person as each body is individual, having its own particular resonance, frequency and energy pattern. Nor does every method of choosing necessarily apply. People perceive energies in different ways. So, you may be kinaesthetic (feeling orientated), intuitive, or logical. If you are logical and head-orientated, you'll probably prefer an issue or intention-matching approach whereas if you are feeling-orientated you'll prefer using your intuition or dowsing. If you're kinaesthetic, it'll be the *feel* of the crystal and what it does to your body and energy field that will help you decide. So try out the methods that appeal to you.

You could, for instance, look up the healing qualities of a crystal or your purpose or symptom (see *Crystal Prescriptions volumes 1* and *2* or *The Crystal Bibles volumes 1–3*). You could use a specific colour of crystal either because of its vibratory effect (see page 23) or a chakra connection (see page 76 and the directory pages). You could look up crystals for your specific requirements (see the A-Z index or the *Crystal Prescriptions* A-Z series). Or, you could match the vibration of a crystal with the type of healing you are undertaking: physical, mental, emotional, spiritual and so on (see below and *Judy Hall's Crystal Companion*). These are examples of an issue or intention-matching process that uses logic and intellect.

You could also choose by diving your hands into a bowl of crystals to see what 'sticks', or allow your eyes to linger on a crystal in a crystal shop or in your own collection. This, together with dowsing, is an intuitive method that utilises your body's extrasensory *knowing* and your inner guidance.

If you dislike a crystal… underlying issues

A clear 'no' response may mean exactly that. The crystal is unsuited to your energy field and needs. However, be aware that your own innate and unconscious reaction to a crystal may, wittingly or unwittingly, affect your choice. Being particularly averse to a crystal at first sight, feeling nauseous when handling it, or getting an exaggerated 'no' or 'panicked' reaction when dowsing, may, unless you are exceptionally well shielded and particularly skilled in the method, indicate that the crystal could treat an underlying issue of which your subconscious (subliminal) mind is aware but which your conscious mind is blocking or repressing. This is particularly so if the issue is karmic or ancestral. You will then instinctively shy away from that crystal, although it may be exactly what you need. Dowsing, or your intuition, may reveal the underlying issue but the beauty of crystal essences is that, if you trust your crystals, the essence will work on an issue *whether you are aware of it or not*.

Essences often work in sequences, one after another. That is to say, you may need to strip away the layers until you reach the core. Each layer requiring a different crystal essence. The final essence in the sequence then transmutes the issue and rebuilds your energy field to an improved and enhanced pattern that will ensure well-being. This sequencing can be approached in one of two ways: taking the essences over a period of days, weeks or months. Or, concatenation in which gem water is taken over a period of hours or days to clear away the layer and then the crystal essence is taken for as long as appropriate (see page 70).

Crystal vibrations

With vibrational frequencies that range from deep and earthy ('lower') to exceedingly fine and cosmic ('higher'), crystals work at many levels: physical, emotional, mental, karmic, ancestral, spiritual, environmental and so on. 'Higher' and 'lower' are not judgemental terms. No one vibration is better than another. Each has their function. It's a matter of vibrational scale. 'Higher' is a much finer, lighter vibration than 'earthy', which functions closer to the earth's vibration. Each has a specific application. There is no point in using an extremely high vibration crystal, which reaches multidimensions and the multiverse, to treat a physical or emotional state. High vibration crystals assist the higher chakras and spiritual imbalances. Some crystals combine both ends of the spectrum, assimilating and grounding higher vibrations into the physical plane. It is through these varied vibrations that remedies made from crystals interact with the physical and subtle bodies, your soul and spirit, and the environment to restore balance.

Earthy (lower/grounding) vibration
The lowest and densest frequency of vibrational resonances, earthy crystals act in the physical world, grounding and anchoring energies. They are protective, detoxifying, cleansing and transmutational. Dense vibration crystals soak up negative energies, transmute them, and transmit beneficial vibes. This is the resonance

of pragmatic concerns, the body and physical well-being, home, safe space, prosperity, material possessions. It brings things into manifestation. A seed vibration of inspiration, fertilisation and creativity; the earthy vibration kickstarts new projects as well as grounding matters into everyday reality. Earthy crystals carry an abundant supply of life force. They resonate with the base, earth star and Gaia gateway chakras to hold you gently in incarnation. These are useful crystals for 'airheads', people who live in the world of ideas and possibilities, or those who only have a toehold in incarnation and find physical reality challenging. Earthy crystals channel energy from planet Earth throughout the whole chakra system to energize and activate all levels of life. Crystals such as Flint or Smoky Quartz carry extremely earthy vibrations.

High vibration

Operating at exceedingly refined multidimensional, 'cosmic' resonances beyond the physicality of Earth, high vibration crystals work at the level of spirit and soul, channelling cosmic energies to earth. The effects 'filter down' into the physical. Cosmic vibration crystals assist spiritual well-being, channelling higher consciousness to Earth. They take you into unity consciousness and universal love, assisting you to accessing your soul's plan and the Akashic Record. High vibe crystals facilitate the ability to be in several dimensions at once. They open the highest crown chakras to reach way up into multidimensions and the multiverse, and activate the causal vortex, soul star and stellar gateway portals, and the alta major chakra within the skull. Many of the 'new' Quartz crystals available today have extremely high vibrations.

Healing vibration

Covering a wide spectrum of energetic resonances, healing vibration crystals are holistic, returning you to a harmonious whole. Crystals combining high vibrations with earthy resonances are effective on the physical plane, promoting well-being. Well-being is a state of mind rather than a physical condition. These crystals facilitate understanding the psychosomatic effect of the mind, emotions and soul's needs on the physical body. They dissolve underlying causes of dis-ease: spiritual, environmental, karmic, psychological, ancestral, emotional or mental imbalances accrued over many lifetimes. Healing vibration crystals facilitate handling change and adjusting to new circumstances, pointing the way forward. Healing crystals cleanse, energize, align and activate the chakras and facilitate assimilation of higher vibrations into the physical and subtle energy bodies.

Dynamic, energetic tools for transformation and well-being, crystals with combined earthy and high vibrations bridge the frequencies of the earth-plane with cosmic dimensions to integrate dualities, infuse higher consciousness into the everyday, and ensure well-being on every level. They harmonise physical and subtle energy bodies, integrating them with the environment and multidimensions that surround us. These crystals elevate denser vibrations and re-form subtle matter. As they have a near-perfect vibration, they entrain energy – that is, return a state of disorder to order. Combination crystals purify, detoxify and transmute at the energetic level, drawing in earthy or cosmic energies as appropriate, and assimilate new frequencies into a purified, receptive physical body. These crystals unify higher chakras above the crown with the earth star and Gaia gateway chakras, integrating refined frequencies throughout the whole chakra system. Bloodstone and the 'bicoloured' crystals such as Quantum Quattro and Que Sera have profoundly healing vibrations.

Colour vibrations

Each colour has its own unique vibration. Different colours of a basic crystal may exhibit significant disparities in their healing effect because of the specific colour vibration. Aragonite is a prime example of this with colours ranging from earthy brown perfect for earth-healing to ethereal white, pink and blue that take you into expanded consciousness. You can utilise colour vibrations to create a crystal essence that harnesses a particular colour effect.

Chalky white, grey, silver, brown or black: Useful protectors, these crystals anchor and ground the physical body and detoxify negative energies.

Bicolour: Excellent integrators, bicoloured crystals harmonise and unify.

Red: Best used for short periods, red crystals stimulate and strengthen. Activating creativity and revitalising potency, red crystals may overexcite volatile emotions or over-energize the body creating hyper-conditions.

Pink: Ideal for long-term use, gentle pink crystals offer unconditional love, nurture and comfort and are excellent for heart healing. They release grief, calm emotions and facilitate acceptance.

Orange: Less volatile than red and appropriate for longer periods, orange crystals activate and release. Building up supportive energetic structures, orange attracts abundance and stimulates creativity.

Yellow and golden: Active at mental and feeling levels, yellow and golden crystals awaken and organise the mind and energize situations. They rebalance and calm emotions and overcome seasonal disorders.

Green: Perfect for environmental healing and the heart, green crystals calm and rebalance. They sedate energy and pacify emotions.

Blue: Calming and clarifying, blue crystals facilitate communication and self-expression. They ground spiritual energy, and assist intuition and channelling.

Purple, indigo and lilac: Integrating and aligning higher energies, these crystals have powerful spiritual awakening qualities, stimulating service to others. These colours cool overheated energies.

White and clear: Clarifying situations and opening intuition to gain insight, white or clear crystals purify and focus energy. They link to the highest realms of being and expanded spiritual consciousness and then integrate the effects into the body or the earth-plane.

[Extracted from *Judy Hall's Crystal Companion*.]

A word of caution

Certain stones contain trace minerals bound up within their chemical makeup that are *potentially* toxic. This does not mean that the crystals cannot be used for essences or crystal healing, however. Indeed, many potentially toxic crystals have been worn or used thera-peutically for millennia. In the modern day, Klinoptilolith (a Zeolite) is the basis for a powerful chemotherapy drug and Zeolite powder is actually used to *remove* toxicity from the environment, despite Zeolite being labelled as 'toxic'. Essences from these stones should be created by an indirect method that transfers the energy signature without transferring any poten-tially toxic material from the crystal (see page 58 for the indirect method). As you will see, some of these poten-tially 'toxic' crystals such as Ruby or Sapphire have been highly regarded for jewellery for thousands of years. Nevertheless, an essence from these gems should be made by the indirect method especially if it is to be taken internally or rubbed gently on the skin. Essences can also be dispersed around the aura if you would prefer to avoid skin contact.

Much is made by opponents of crystal healing of the dangers of, say, Chrysotile, which contains asbestos. But crystals containing asbestos would need to be rough and frayed in order for any toxic dust to be inhaled, which is impossible if you use a tumbled stone. To avoid the stone would be to reject a powerful karmic healer. Be sensible and exercise caution when handling such crystals, however. Use potentially toxic crystals in a tumbled, faceted or polished form wherever possible. If in doubt, create an essence by the indirect method. This method is also suitable for fragile and delicate crystals; soluble stones, such as Halite or Selenite; or layered stones such as Muscovite. Handle with care and always wash your hands after handling these stones (see the A-Z of Contraindications page 312–318).

Dowsing

Dowsing quickly identifies the right crystal for you. You can either use a pendulum for this purpose or finger, body or rod dowse. Pendulums may spin wildly or sluggishly and will indicate 'yes', 'no' or 'maybe' – in which case ask if there is a crystal that would be more beneficial for your purpose. Muscle testing can also rapidly pinpoint the right crystal for you. There are several methods of dowsing so try them all until you find the one that works best for you and then practise to refine your technique. You will need to establish your 'yes' and 'no' signal if using a pendulum (see below). Dowsing for crystals works best in an energetically clear space so spray an environmental cleansing essence before commencing.

Pendulum dowsing

If you are familiar with pendulum dowsing, use the pendulum in your usual way. If you are not, this skill is easily learned. Crystal pendulums can be used for this but choose something neutral like a Quartz or an Agate so that the crystal's energy does not interfere with your choice. Inert wooden or metal pendulums can also be used.

To pendulum dowse

As with crystals, everyone's response to dowsing varies. To pendulum dowse, hold your pendulum between the thumb and forefinger of your most receptive hand with about a hand's length of chain hanging down to the pendulum – you will soon learn what is the right length for you. Wrap the remaining chain around your fingers so that it does not obstruct the dowsing.

You will need to ascertain which is a 'yes' and which is a 'no' response. Some people find that the pendulum swings in one direction for 'yes' and at right angles to that axis for 'no', while others have a backwards and forwards swing for one reply, and a circular motion for the other. A 'wobble' of the pendulum may indicate a 'maybe' or that it is not appropriate to dowse at that time, or that the wrong question is being asked. In which case, ask if it is appropriate to dowse at that time. If the answer is 'yes', check that you are framing the question in the correct way. If the pendulum stops completely it is usually inappropriate to ask at that time.

You can ascertain your particular pendulum response by holding the pendulum over your knee and asking: "Is my name [correct name]?" The direction that the pendulum swings will indicate 'yes'. Check by asking: "Is my name [incorrect name]?" to establish 'no'. Mix your name up, a true and false name combined to check for 'maybe' or 'Huh?'. Or, you can programme in 'yes' and 'no' by swinging the pendulum in a particular direction a few times, saying as you do: "This is yes" and swinging it in a different direction to programme in 'no'.

Remember that a violent 'no' response or a wild 'figure of eight' swing may be your body's way of telling you that there is an underlying issue or conflict that is causing an aversion to the very stone that may be exactly what you need. Always check it out by further questioning.

To dowse a crystal or list: Once yes or no is established, simply place your finger on a crystal, or its name, or run your finger down an appropriate list and ask, "Is this crystal beneficial for me?" You may identify several possible crystals and need to refine the answer.

Finger Dowsing

Finger dowsing answers 'yes' and 'no' questions quickly and unambiguously and may be done unobtrusively in situations where a pendulum might provoke unwanted attention. This method of dowsing works particularly well for people who are kinaesthetic, that is to say their body responds intuitively to subtle feelings, but anyone can learn to finger dowse.

To finger dowse

To finger dowse, hold the thumb and first finger of your right hand together (see illustration). Loop the thumb and finger of your left hand through to make a 'chain'. Ask your question clearly and unambiguously – you can speak it aloud or keep it within your mind. Now pull gently but firmly. If the chain breaks, the answer is usually 'no'. If it holds, the answer is usually 'yes' – but check by asking your name in case your response is reversed.

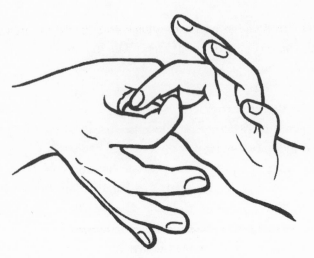

Finger dowsing

To rod dowse

You can use purpose-made dowsing rods, y-shaped hazel twigs or cut wire coat hangers into right-angled shapes to find detrimental energy lines or to pinpoint where to disperse an environmental or aspirational essence. However, it is more difficult to pinpoint a crystal from a list with this method.

Method:

- Hold the rods loosely in your hands, fingers curled inwards to make a holder, and slowly walk forwards across a room or site.
- Ask to be shown where the lines of disturbance or appropriate placement are.
- The rods will move or twitch when you reach the

front edge and move back to straight when you pass beyond it.

Body dowsing

As bodies are extremely sensitive to changing vibrations you could use your hands to select a crystal or your feet to dowse your space.

Dowsing with the palm chakras:

- If you are using your hands rub your hands together briskly to open your palm chakras.
- Then *feel* the energy of the crystal and monitor your response to it. A crystal that will work for you or your space will feel lively, tingly as you pick it up. Place it in your space or on your body and, if your hand then feels calm, this is the crystal for you. A crystal that feels 'dead' and lifeless will do nothing for you. A crystal that burns or jumps may be exactly the right crystal for you but may need to be used in conjunction with a regulating crystal to direct the energy (see page 52).
- Similarly, if you hold your hand palm down over a chakra and it is blocked, it will feel lifeless or sticky. If it is whirling too fast, you will feel a strong and uncomfortable buzzing in your palm. Choose an appropriate crystal to create an essence to restore the energy to optimum.

Muscle testing

Another method that utilises body dowsing is to muscle test.

To muscle test:

- Extend the arm that you use to write with out sideways at shoulder height.
- With the other hand, hold a crystal over a chakra or over the centre of your chest.
- Ask a friend to stand behind you and press down on your extended arm at the wrist, saying, "Resist."
- If the arm remains strong and firm, this is the right crystal for you. If the arm drops, try another crystal.

Feeling crystal energy

If you are kinaesthetic your body responds to energy in ways that may include jerking, twitching, a sensation as though icy water is running down your spine, or your belly getting hot, your head or hands buzzing and the like. You may feel dizzy or nauseous, or on a high. You can easily check out how you respond to a particular crystal:

To sense crystal energy:

- Rub your hands together to activate your palm chakras.
- Hold the crystal and breathe gently letting the

energy flow from the crystal into your hands and
up your arms.

- Monitor your body to see how it responds. Move it
up the chakras if you feel this is appropriate.
- The strongest response, positive or 'negative', will
indicate a crystal that could work for you
especially if there is an underlying issue that
requires healing.

Purifying and focusing your crystals

Purifying your crystals

As crystals hold the energetic charge of everyone who comes into contact with them and rapidly absorb emanations from their surroundings as well as your personal energies they need purifying on a regular basis. It is sensible to cleanse and re-energize a crystal every time it is used for an essence. The method employed will depend on the type of crystal. Soft, layered and friable crystals, for instance, and those that are attached to a matrix base may be damaged by water or frost. Soft stones such as Halite (a salt) or Selenite will dissolve. These are best purified by a 'dry' process such as brown rice and recharged by sun or moon light. Sturdier crystals benefit from being held under running water (preferably not tap water) or in the sea.

Methods:

Running water

Hold your crystals in running water, or pour bottled water over them, or place in them a stream or the ocean to draw off negative energy (use a bag to hold small crystals). You could also immerse appropriate crystals in a bowl of water into which a handful of sea salt or rock salt has been added. (Salt is best avoided if the crystal is layered or friable, however.) Dry the crystal carefully afterwards and place in the sun to re-energize or use a proprietary crystal recharging essence.

Returning to the earth

You will need to dowse to establish the length of time a crystal needs to return to the earth in order to cleanse and recharge as the period will differ with each crystal. If you do not have a garden, a flowerpot filled with soil or sand can be used instead. If you bury crystals to cleanse them, remember to mark the spot.

Rice

Place your crystal in a bowl of rice overnight, and then afterward compost the rice (do not eat it). Brown rice seems to have a special affinity with crystals that have been subjected to EMF or negative energy pollution, rapidly drawing it off. Place the crystals in the sun or under the moon to re-energize if appropriate or use a crystal essence (see page 68 and Resources).

Salt

Salt – and Halite – also draws off toxic energies but may be damaging to layered or friable crystals. If using salt, brush it off carefully and make sure that it has been removed from any niches or cracks in the crystal as otherwise it will absorb water in the future and could cause splintering. Salt is best used in a 'salt-ring' around the crystal.

Crystals

Crystals such as Carnelian, Smoky Quartz or Citrine can cleanse another crystal, but will need cleansing themselves afterwards.

Smudging

Sage, sweetgrass or joss sticks are excellent for smudging as they quickly remove negative energies. Light the smudge stick and pass it over the crystal if it is large, or hold the crystal in your hand in the smoke if it is small. It is traditional to fan the smoke gently with a feather but this is not essential.

Sound

Sound tuning forks, bells, tingshaws, a Tibetan bowl or gong over the crystal to cleanse it and then recharge in sun or moon light.

Visualising light

Hold your crystal in your hands and visualise a column of bright white light coming down and covering the crystal, absorbing anything negative it may have picked up and restoring the pure energy once more. If you find visualisation difficult, you can use the light of a candle. Crystals also respond well to being placed in sun or moon light to cleanse and recharge.

Crystal clearing essences

A number of crystal and space clearing essences are

available from essence suppliers, crystal shops and the Internet (see Resources). Personally I never move far without Petaltone Clear2Light, a crystal and space clearing essence, and Petaltone Z14, an etheric clearer. You can either drop the essence directly on to the crystal, gently rubbing it over the crystal with your finger, or put a few drops into clean spring water in an atomiser or spray bottle and gently mist the crystal. However, you can also create your own clearing essence:

Crystal cleansing and recharging essence

Choose one or two from each list and combine:

Cleansing/Clearing crystals: Black Tourmaline, Blue or Black Kyanite, Citrine (natural), Halite, Hanksite, Hematite, Shungite, Smoky Quartz

Recharging: Anandalite™, Carnelian, Citrine, Golden Healer, Orange Kyanite, Quartz, Red Jasper, Selenite

To create the essence:

- Hold the crystals in your hands and ask them to cleanse your crystals or space.
- Place all the crystals in a glass bowl and pour on spring water (note: although Selenite or Halite is soluble, place them directly in water for this particular essence). Remove the crystals and pour the essence into a large glass bottle. Add a few drops of essential oil such as frankincense, sage or lavender if liked and top up with two-thirds vodka

or white rum unless the essence is to be used for addictions, in which case choose another preservative. This is the mother essence. Label bottle with date and contents. Keep in a cool place.

To use: Fill a spray bottle with spring water. Add seven drops of mother essence. Lightly mist crystals or space.

Recharging your crystal

Crystals can be placed on a Quartz cluster, 'bed' (a flat piece covered in small crystals) or within a geode, or on a large Carnelian to re-energize them. Or, you can use a proprietary crystal recharger (Petaltone and The Crystal Balance Company make excellent ones, see Resources) but the light of the sun is a natural energizer. Red and yellow crystals particularly enjoy being placed in the sun, and white and pale-coloured crystals respond well to the full moon. (Be aware that sunlight focused through a crystal may be a fire hazard and delicate crystals will lose their colour quickly if left exposed to light.) Some brown crystals, such as Smoky Quartz, respond to being placed on or in the earth to recharge. If you bury a crystal, remember to mark its position clearly.

Focusing and activating your crystal

Crystals work best when their energy is harnessed and focused with intent towards the task at hand as this activates them. By taking the time to attune a crystal to your own unique frequency, you enhance its vibratory effect and amplify its healing power.

Method:

- Once your crystal has been purified and re-energized, sit quietly holding the crystal in your hands for a few minutes until you feel in tune with it.
- Picture it surrounded by light and love. State that the crystal is dedicated to the highest good of all who use it.
- Then state clearly your intention for the crystal – that it will heal or protect you, for instance, or that it will transmute negative energy.
- If the essence is intended for a specific purpose, state that also. Repeat the intention several times to anchor it into the crystal.

Deprogramming a crystal

There may be times when a crystal has been dedicated for one particular use but is no longer required for that purpose. This does not mean its usefulness is over. Far from it; it will undoubtedly have other work to do and another purpose to carry out. The crystal should be deprogrammed, cleansed and rededicated before reuse especially when creating an essence.

As has been seen, crystals hold thoughts and intentions. Which means that if you have been gifted a crystal, whatever the giver envisioned or intended for you will be programmed into the crystal. Similarly, the crystal may be automatically imprinted with assumptions as to what that crystal does. The labels in a crystal shop or a description on the Internet is sufficient to do that. The deepest intention someone has may be unconscious and unacknowledged – and far from what they thought they were putting into a crystal. It is therefore sensible to thoroughly deprogramme a crystal and put your own intention into it before use in an essence.

However, crystals can also be used to create a 'defragging essence' that removes previous programming (see below):

To deprogramme a crystal

- Hold the crystal in your hands for a few moments, thanking it for doing its work and for holding the intention and purpose it has had. Explain to the crystal that this part of its work is now over and ask the crystal to dismantle the programme it has been carrying.

- See bright white light beaming into the crystal to help it to deprogramme, cleanse and recharge.
- Wash the crystal in Clear2Light and/or Z14 or other cleansing essence (see page 41), or place it under running water.
- Put the crystal out into sunlight for a few hours or under the moon.
- The crystal may need a rest period to rebuild its energies before being rededicated to a new purpose.

If you are non-visual: Cleanse the crystal with Clear2Light or your own purpose-made clearing essence, place it under running water or into brown rice, and then into sun or moon light. Then place the crystal on a Brandenberg Quartz – or if the crystal is large, place the Brandenberg on the crystal – and ask that it be returned to its original, pure programme and purpose. Leave overnight. Then remove the crystal and allow it to rest before being rededicated.

Deprogramming crystal essence

This essence is particularly useful when a crystal has been in use for one particular purpose for a long time but it can also remove programming and intention from a crystal no matter what the source. It can also be helpful for removing the final remnants of deeply ingrained programming within the physical or subtle bodies, or within the environment.

- Select your crystals from the 'defragging crystal list' below and create an essence by the direct method (see page 58).
- Drop the essence on to the crystal that is to be deprogrammed and leave it in the sun to recharge, or spray with a recharging essence (see page 41).

'Defragging' crystals: Anandalite, Ancestralite, Brandenberg Amethyst, Celtic Quartz, Cradle of Life (Humanity), Freedom Stone, Golden Lemurian Seed, Iolite-and-Sunstone, Lapis Lace, Lazulite-spotted Blue Quartz, Rainbow Lattice Sunstone, Rainbow Mayanite, Sea Foam Flint, Strawberry Lemurian Seed, Temple Calcite.

Part III

Creating a crystal essence

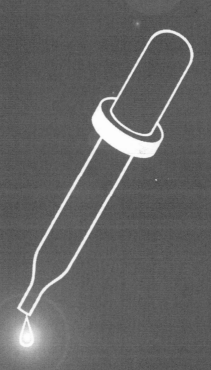

Before you begin

As crystals pick up the vibes from the environment around them and from a person handling them, a few simple precautions ensure that only beneficial energies transfer to the essence you are preparing (see Purifying your crystals page 38). Your frame of mind is crucial. The 'observer/participant effect' has been scientifically observed for many years so be aware that your mood – and that of anyone around you – may beneficially or adversely affect the outcome. Cynicism, disbelief or rubbishing the idea will prejudicially affect an essence. As will having a rigidly fixed outcome or expectation in mind. Crystals have an innate intelligence that ascertains what is required and cooperates with your intuition – if you allow it. An essence may well do more than you believed possible, so always allow for that possibility by keeping an open mind.

Water too can pick up the vibrations of your thoughts and tap water may be polluted with 'decontaminants' or hormones. So it is sensible to use spring water, ensuring that it has not been contaminated with fertiliser, and to be in the best possible frame of mind before handling the water.

A few tips:

- Begin an essence when you are in a positive frame of mind.
- Never begin an essence when you are feeling

fearful, depressed or angry.

- Shield yourself with a protective crystal or aura spray (see page 51).
- Centre and ground yourself before beginning.
- Cleanse your crystals immediately before placing them in the bowl.
- Work with a clear intention and without expectation as to the outcome.

Centring and grounding

Grounding is a term that means you are solidly anchored in the present, with a certain inner stillness, a feeling of being secure, in control of yourself and alert.
– Simon Lilly, *Crystals & Crystal Healing*

This simple grounding root exercise anchors you to the planet, re-energizes you from the Earth, and centres you in your body before creating an essence. It is worth doing any time you are going to work with crystals, essences or vibrational healing energies. After awhile it becomes second nature and only takes a minute or so. Remember to cleanse and dedicate your crystals before you begin the exercise (see pages 38–43).

Creating a grounding root:

- Cleanse your aura and chakras by passing Flint and/or Anandalite around your body. (If you don't have Anandalite or the other crystals you can use the cards in *The Crystal Wisdom Healing Oracle* pack.) Or, spray your aura with an aura cleansing essence followed by a centring essence (see below).

- Stand with your feet slightly apart, well balanced on your knees and hips. Feet flat on the floor. Place a Flint, Eye of the Storm (Judy's Jasper), Graphic Smoky Quartz, Hematite, Smoky Quartz, Smoky Quartz Elestial or other grounding stone at your feet. Or, rub a grounding essence on the soles of your feet.

- Picture the earth star chakra about a foot beneath your feet opening like the petals of a water lily.

- Place your hands just below your navel (tummy button) with fingertips touching and palms out towards the hips.

- Picture roots spreading across your belly, into your hips and then down through your legs and out of your feet to meet in the grounding stone.

- The two roots twine together and pass down through the earth star and the Gaia gateway, going deep into the earth. They pass through the outer mantle, down past the solid crust and deep into the molten magma.

- When the entwined roots have passed through the magma, they reach the big iron crystal ball at the centre of the planet.

- The roots hook themselves around this ball, holding you firmly in incarnation and helping you to be grounded in incarnation.

- Energy and protection can flow up this root to keep you energized and safe.
- Allow the roots to pass up from the earth star through your feet, up your legs and the knee chakras and into your hips. At your hips the roots move across to meet in the base chakra and from there to the sacral and the dantien just below your navel. The energy that flows up from the centre of the Earth can be stored in the dantien, the centre of gravity for your physical body.

Centring essence: Bloodstone, Calcite, Celestobarite, Coral*, Eye of the Storm (Judy's Jasper), Flint, Fossilised Wood, Gaia's Blood Flint, Garnet, Grape Chalcedony, Hematite, Kunzite, Obsidian, Onyx, Peanut Wood, Prairie Tanzanite, Quartz, Red Jasper, Ruby, Sardonyx, Shiva Lingam, Tourmalinated Quartz. *Chakra:* Gaia gateway, earth star, base, dantien

Grounding essence: Apache Tear, Black Tourmaline, Eye of the Storm (Judy's Jasper), Flint, Granite with Garnet or Ruby, Graphic Smoky Quartz, Hematite, Master Shamanite, Shungite, Smoky Quartz, Smoky Quartz Elestial

*Always use ethically sourced Coral that has not been obtained from a living reef.

Regulatory crystals

If you are a particularly sensitive, or energetically depleted, person or suffer from a chronic condition, you may need to add regulatory crystals to an essence to ensure that it works slowly and gently, allowing your body and psyche to respond at the pace that is right for you, or that it speeds up sluggish energy assimilation. Similarly if your chakras are over or under active, a regulatory crystal will ensure that the essence stimulates or sedates the chakra as appropriate. Either include the regulatory crystal in the mix, or in the case of soluble crystals such as Halite and Selenite, stand the crystal alongside the bowl during essence creation if you prefer.

Regulatory crystals: Aragonite, Black Kyanite, Brandenberg Amethyst, Calcite, Charoite, Chromium Quartz, Fluorite, Grape Chalcedony, Green Kyanite, Halite, Isua, Kiwi Stone (Sesame Jasper), Ocean Jasper, Prairie Tanzanite, Quartz, Rose Quartz, Selenite, Serpentine, Shungite, Smoky Quartz, Tanzurine (Cherry and Emerald Quartz)

Timing: full, new moon, solstice, equinox, eclipse, etc.

Most essences can be created as and when required or when an opportunity arises. The mother essence will keep for years if sufficient alcohol or other preservative is added. Having said that, however, if the mother or dosage bottle essence begins to smell 'off', with a mouldy tang, or if it develops sediment in the bottom or goes cloudy, throw it away (with the exception of Shungite Water which, when made by the direct method, will always have fine black particulates suspended within it).

Other essences take on the astronomical conditions at the time they are created, cosmic events reinforcing the vibrations. Some amazing essences can be created by timing their inception with the full, new moon, solstices, equinoxes, eclipses and so on. White crystals are particularly sensitive to the moon's fluctuating cycle, and yellow crystals love to work with the sun's passage around the zodiac and with lunar eclipses. Dark crystals gestate in the dark of the moon and respond to solar eclipses. The Moon can take on different shades of red, orange or gold during a total lunar eclipse and crystals with these colours also respond more strongly at this time.

If you are dealing with ancestral or karmic issues, then an essence created during an eclipse will allow previously repressed factors to rise up for resolution. If you are dealing with paternal issues, then an essence created during an eclipse of the sun ameliorates a strong authoritarian influence to create equilibrium between the parental influences. Similarly if you are dealing with maternal issues, a lunar eclipse bypasses 'the great-no-sayer' influence of a powerful mother-figure and reveals the previously hidden, but equally potent, effect of a weakened father-figure. The essence would then bring the two influences into balance.

You'll find further calendrical, cosmic and planetary connections in the astrological section to assist timing your essence creating (see page 141).

Creating an Essence

Equipment required

One or two glass bowls according to the method
selected

Funnel

Glass bottle for storage

Spring water

Alcohol or other preservative

Appropriate crystals

Dosage dropper bottle or spray

Water

Spring water should be used for essences rather than tap
water that potentially has chlorine, fluoride and
aluminium added to it and which may carry hormones
or toxic residues. If you must use tap water, pass it
through a commercial filter first. Water from a spring
with healing properties is particularly effective provided
it is from an uncontaminated source.

Sterilising your equipment

Even if you are creating gem water for immediate consumption, it is sensible to use sterile equipment whenever possible – although I have made flower and essences of place 'in the field' while on holiday, using my water bottle or other drinks bottle. Whatever is to hand as you never quite know when you'll come across an opportunity. If I have to use a plastic bottle, which I prefer to avoid, I transfer the essence to a glass bottle once one's available. Boil your equipment before you begin, or use colloidal silver, Citricidal, or Shungite Water to ensure there are no bacteria, viruses or fungi to contaminate the process. This is also a time when microwaves can be useful. A minute or two in a microwave sterilises a glass bottle and removes the vibratory memory of any previous contents.

Sprays or dropper bottles

You will need a reasonable-sized glass bottle in which to store your mother essence. Coloured glass is preferable to clear as it preserves the vibrations better. The essence can then be transferred to a dosage dropper or spray bottle as required. These bottles can be purchased in chemists or drugstores or via the Internet. If reusing a bottle, remember to sterilise it and remove the vibratory memory.

Direct and indirect preparation methods

There are two distinct methods of preparing essences. One is direct. Crystals are immersed in the spring water and placed in the sun – or on a crystal cluster if there is no prospect of sunlight for awhile. This method is suitable for non-toxic and non-friable or non-soluble crystals. Sound can also be used to transfer the vibration to the water – some powerful essences have been made in Tibetan bowls for instance. Or, you can steep your crystals in a pure carrier oil and use it for massage.

The second method is the bowl-within-a-bowl indirect method or bowl-on-a-photograph, which can also be combined with sound. In the indirect method, the crystals do not have direct contact with the water. Large crystals can also be placed next to a bowl of water and the vibrations transferred either by contact with the bowl or by sound. The water stores the crystal energy-pattern-vibrations and transfers them to the physical or subtle bodies, the environment or the planet.

Crystal tip: Do remember that, if a crystal is rare or expensive, you can always add a few drops of the mother essence of that crystal (so that you only have to make it once) to a future essence. You do not have to use the crystal itself. The Crystal Balance Company (see Resources) makes crystal essences from rare crystals and these can be added to your crystal mix. You can also use a photograph to transfer the crystal vibes (see below).

Direct method

- Place enough spring water in a glass bowl to just cover the crystal.
- If there is no prospect of sunlight, stand the bowl on a large Quartz crystal cluster or bed, or within a geode. Clear Quartz, Citrine or Amethyst work well.
- Stand the bowl in sunlight (or on the cluster) for several hours. (If the bowl is left outside, cover with a glass lid or cling film to prevent insects falling into it.)
- If appropriate, the bowl can also be left overnight in moonlight.
- The essence is now ready to be preserved and bottled as per bottling and storage below.

Indirect method

- If the crystal is potentially toxic, soluble or fragile (see Contraindications page 311) place the crystal in a small glass bowl and stand the bowl within a large bowl that has sufficient spring water to raise the level above the crystal in the inner bowl.
- Stand the bowl in sunlight, or on a crystal cluster, for several hours. (If the bowl is left outside, cover

with a glass lid or cling film.)

- If appropriate, the bowl can also be left overnight in moonlight.
- Large crystals can be placed touching the bowl to transfer the vibrations.
- The essence is now ready to be preserved and bottled as per bottling and storage below.

Sound method

As sound is also a vibration it assists with the rapid transfer of crystal vibrations into water. This method is especially efficient where an 'instant' essence is required, or when there is no sun available to 'set' the essence. A variety of instruments can be used according to those you have at hand or your intuition tells you would be appropriate. Indigenous instruments are particularly effective. Crystals from Australia respond well to a didgeridoo and those from the Himalayas to a Tibetan bowl or tingshaws.

Example: On a workshop for soul midwives in training, for instance, when exploring crystals to assist with death and transition I took along a large Trigonic Quartz. Trigonic Quartz holds the record of a soul's journey from its commencement as it leaves the initial pool of soul essence to wherever the end may be way out in the 'future' (although time has little meaning outside the earth-plane). Trigonic is an Akashic Recordkeeper with each crystal linking holistically to the whole. A Trigonic is rare and expensive so it would not be an easy crystal for individuals to purchase (but see crystal supplier recommendations in Resources section). We wanted to create a mother tincture that each participant could take away with them. We had limited time in which to create an essence so decided on sound as that was a tool the soul midwives already used to assist transition. We took a large Tibetan bowl and placed the Trigonic in the centre of the water and gently struck the bowl with a beater. The effect was extraordinary. Myriad triangles radiated out from the crystal across the surface of the water. The identifying factor for a Trigonic is upside-down triangles cascading down the crystal. The essence creation was instant and it could be bottled immediately. It was extremely effective in facilitating gentle transition to the next world.

Sound Method:

- Stand the cleansed crystal in a Tibetan or glass bowl and cover with spring water. Or place in a bowl-within-a-bowl of water if the crystal contains toxic elements or is friable. Large crystals can be placed alongside a metal bowl of water.
- If using a Tibetan or metal bowl, gently tap the side of the bowl with a beater or play the bowl by drawing a beater or violin bow around the rim.
- If using a drum, tingshaw or tuning fork, sound it over the bowl.
- If using a didgeridoo, sound it across the surface of

the water.

- The essence is now ready to be preserved and bottled as per bottling and storage below.

The photographic method

Some crystals are extremely rare and difficult to obtain. But all is not lost if you cannot obtain the actual crystal. High quality, high resolution photographs, such as those in my *Crystal Wisdom Healing Oracle*, *101 Power Crystals*, *Crystal Companion* or on my website www.judyhall.co.uk – where I post photographs of the latest crystals – can be utilised as a skilled, energetically aware, photographer can capture the crystal's vibrations in a digital photograph. Photographs of crystals such as Ancestralite, Anandalite, Brandenberg Amethyst, Rainbow Mayanite, Lapis Lace, Strawberry or Golden Lemurian Seed, Iolite-and-Sunstone, Rainbow Lattice Sunstone, Sea Foam Flint or Cradle of Life are perfect for this method. Once an essence is created, a few drops can be added to future essences where required to remove the last remnants of an inappropriate energy pattern or to introduce a higher-dimensional-consciousness vibration.

Method:

- Place the photograph under or alongside a bowl of spring water and proceed as for the indirect method.
- Bottle the mother essence and then add a few drops of the mother essence (see below) without

further dilution when required for deep-seated issue essences.

Bottling and preserving

If a crystal essence is not to be used within a day or two, top up with two-thirds brandy, vodka, white rum, cider vinegar or other preservative to one-third essence, otherwise the essence will become musty. The ancients used honey, which is antibacterial and the modern equivalent could perhaps be mead, which is made from fermented honey. You could also add a small piece of Shungite as this is antibacterial, antiviral and antifungal. This creates a 'mother essence' that will keep for years and which is further diluted.

I return any unused short-term essence or leftover water from the first creation stage as a libation to give thanks to the earth. Pouring it either directly on the earth, a rock, or in a flowing stream. Where appropriate I also use it to nourish my pot plants or to cleanse and strengthen the properties of my crystals.

Preservatives: Brandy, Cider Vinegar, Citricidal, Glycerol, Mead, Shungite, Vodka, White Rum

Essential oils: frankincense, lavender, myrrh, sage

Storage

Once you have made the mother essence, label it and then store it in a cool, dark place. Wherever possible, place bottles with space around them. Dosage strengths, however, can be kept in a cupboard, your pocket or a handbag depending on how often you are using the essence. If a mother or dosage bottle essence or a spray begins to smell 'off' with a mouldy tang, or if it develops sediment in the bottom or goes cloudy, throw it away (with the exception of Shungite Water which, when made by the direct method, will always have fine black particulates suspended within it).

Stock and dosage bottles

Traditionally, a stock bottle is then prepared using one-third brandy or other preservative to two-thirds spring water and seven drops of mother essence are added. This is further diluted to make a small dosage bottle; add seven drops of the mother essence to a dosage bottle containing two-thirds water and one-third brandy. If a spray bottle is being made, add seven drops of mother essence to pure water if using immediately. For prolonged use, vodka or white rum make useful preservatives in spray bottles as they have no smell; essential oils can also be added although, in time, these may clog sprays and droppers.

Alternative methods

These methods are based on ancient procedures that can be equally effective today.

Carrier oil

A good quality, preferably organic, massage oil base can be utilised to create a crystal massage oil. You can blend several compatible crystals into the mix.

You will need:

Good quality massage carrier oil

Appropriate crystals

Bowl(s) and bottle for mother essence

Small glass jug or wide-necked jar with stopper

Essential oils if appropriate

Spring water

Crystal cluster, flat crystal bed or geode if appropriate

Steeping method:

- Pour the oil into a small, glass jug or wide-necked jar.
- Place the selected crystals into the oil. Stopper the neck or cover the top.
- Place in sunlight if possible – a windowsill can be utilised.
- Steep the crystals in the oil for an appropriate length of time (dowse to establish length).
- Add a few drops of essential oil if appropriate.

- Bottle the oil in a dark-coloured glass bottle with a screw top when dowsing indicates it is ready for use. You can add small chips or tumbled crystals into the bottle if the essence is going to be kept for some time. But ensure that these do not tip out of the bottle into your hand when using the oil for massage.

Carrier cream

A few drops of an appropriate mother essence can also be worked into a neutral, non-fragranced, aqueous-cream base for application to the skin. Essences can also be added to manuka honey, a natural antibiotic, to assist wound healing.

Gem water

Gem water is made for immediate use utilising water and sun and/or moonlight. As they are not preserved, the energy transfer is short term and the essence must be used within hours of its creation. Many gems are potentially toxic (see Contraindications) and, in such cases, gem water should be made using the indirect method.

- Place the crystal in pure spring water in a glass bowl (or a bowl-within-a-bowl) and leave in sunlight or moonlight for several hours, or place on to a crystal bed. Cover the bowl with cling film if left outside.
- Use immediately.

Shungite Water

Shungite Water is, in effect, a crystal essence. But it does not require diluting nor does it require a preservative. Shungite water has been shown by research to remove harmful elements such as bacteria and free radicals, and to support your immune system. To become biologically active, water needs to have Shungite immersed in it for at least forty-eight hours. However, once the first batch is made, simply refill the filter jug every time you use some of the water so that it is constantly replenished. Wash the filter jug and the bag of Shungite at least once a week depending on how much water you have used (you can store the activated water and return it to the jug). Place the Shungite in the sun or air for a few hours to recharge, or alternate two bags. Raw Shungite is more effective than the tumbled, but, no matter how often the non-vitreous type of Shungite has been washed, it does tend to leave a very fine suspension of black particles in the water. This is harmless and part of the process. However, if you prefer, and if you are using Elite or Noble Shungite, the essence can be made by the indirect method. *Note: although most filter jugs are plastic, the Shungite appears to overcome this.*

You will need:

2 litre filter jug
Water, preferably spring but if using tap water pass it through a commercial filter first

Fine mesh 2″ bag of raw Shungite (10–100gm) or a small glass container of Shungite if creating by the indirect method

Creating the water:

- Place the mesh bag or glass bottle of Shungite in the base of the filter jug (if using tap water you use a commercial filter if the jug is provided with one).
- Pour water into the jug until it is full.
- Stand it aside for 48 hours.
- Then top up the water each time it is used.
- Cleanse the Shungite frequently under running water and re-energize in the sun or air.

Wine or Mead

The ancients added crystals to mead or to wine, or to juices such as pomegranate – now being recognised as a 'superfood', with antioxidant and various other healing properties. In some cases, 'vigorous boiling' was the recommended method of preparation, in others steeping. It is worth experimenting to see which works for you. It is not necessary to pulverise the crystal. The vibrations will transfer and bring about healing from the whole crystal.

Using your crystal essences

Essences convey crystal vibes to the body or the environment at a subtle level, repatterning your cells to optimum. Many of the directory entries indicate a chakra link through which a condition can be healed or a chakra balanced, or you can dowse for or intuit this (see page 31, and *Crystal Prescriptions 4* for further information on the physiology of the chakras). One way to take a crystal essence is through a dosage bottle, from which you take seven drops by mouth, or on the skin or in your bathwater. Most essences can be sprayed around the aura or over clothing on the chakra, or over organs or the site of dis-ease; or be rubbed directly on to the skin. You can also use the concatenation – sequential – method below (see page 70).

Using a crystal essence, oils or gem water

- Essences intended for adult use can, where appropriate, be taken directly into the mouth from a dosage bottle, or be added to a glass of water and sipped.
- Essences for children can be gentled rubbed on the wrist or dropped into bathwater.
- A few drops of an essence can be gently rubbed on appropriate chakras. Dowse to check how many applications are necessary.
- For both adults and young people, essences can be

applied to the palm chakras and then swept all around the aura (about an arm's length out from the body). Remember to sweep behind the body as well as the front and sides. This is particularly useful when using protection essences.

- For short-term use, an essence can be sipped every few minutes or rubbed on the affected part. Hold the water in your mouth for a few moments. If a dropper bottle has been made, drop seven drops under your tongue at regular intervals until the symptoms or condition ceases.

- Essences can also be applied to the skin, either at the wrist or over the site of a problem, or added to bathwater.

- If a spray bottle is made, spray all around the aura or around the room taking care to spray into corners and under furniture. This is particularly effective for clearing negative energies, especially from the crystals themselves, or from a sickroom or an electromagnetically or emotionally stressed place.

- When you have taken, sprayed, dispersed or rubbed in the essence, close your eyes, breathe gently and evenly, and allow yourself to relax and feel the energy of the crystal radiating out through your whole being or your environment. Hold the intention that the stones will work for you.

- Essences can also be 'breathed in' by applying them to the palms of your hands and then, with your hands to your nose, inhaling deeply.

- If using gem water, drink immediately when the glass has been prepared.
- If using Shungite Water, drink several glasses a day, topping up the water in the filter jug as you draw it off.
- If massaging with a crystal oil, it is preferable to leave the oil on the skin to be absorbed rather than showering it off immediately after the massage.

Concatenation

Concatenation means sequencing crystal energies in order to strip back superficial and then progressively deeper layers to reach and rebalance the core of a problem or issue. The need for concatenation is indicated by a large number of crystals receiving a strong 'yes' indication *even after you have asked, "Is this crystal necessary or is there one that will be more appropriate/beneficial/efficient?"* Choose a day when you will not be disturbed for several hours.

Method:

- If your dowsing, or other method of choosing crystals, has revealed a larger number than four crystals, arrange them in single or group piles according to the sequence in which you dowse or intuit they should be utilised.
- Check which of the piles is to be used to create a crystal essence and prepare the mother essence by

an appropriate method (see above) preserving it in brandy or other preservative. Set the mother essence aside.

- Check the order in which the remaining crystals are to be utilised.
- Place the first crystal(s) into half a glass of spring water. Either place the glass in sunlight or on to a crystal bed for five to ten minutes, or gently use sound to transfer the vibrations.
- Drink immediately.
- Wait quietly.
- When a suitable interval has passed – dowse, intuit or wait for a response or reaction to subside – create and take the next gem water in the sequence.
- Continue taking gem waters until you reach the final essence, allowing yourself plenty of time. DON'T OVERDO IT. If traumatic memories or ingrained layers of resistance are being released, you may need to do this process over several days or even weeks. Always allow a response to subside before taking or applying the next crystal in the sequence.
- When you reach the final stage, dilute the mother essence that you created at the beginning of the process into a dosage bottle (see page 56).
- Take or apply seven drops three times a day for as long as appropriate – your intuition, 'symptoms' subsiding, or 'the process is complete' dowsing

response will let you know when to stop taking the essence. Often you find that you slowly tail off by 'forgetting' to take the essence. This is an excellent indication that the process is coming to an end.

Distant use of essences

Distant healing is possible with permission of the recipient. Place a photograph or the name of the recipient where it will not be disturbed. Place a Quartz crystal over it. Drop the essence on several times a day. Alternatively, if you are an experienced energy practitioner, you can use your own body as a surrogate for the recipient, placing the essence on your own body or around your aura whilst holding the recipient strongly in mind.

How often?

In acute situations, essences can be sipped or rubbed on every half an hour or so, but in less acute situations two or three times a day is usually sufficient. Sprays are used as and when required.

Healing challenge

Occasionally an essence, especially when used for space clearing or toxicity release, or where there is an underlying condition, will trigger a 'healing challenge' where the symptoms appear to get worse rather than better and flu-like symptoms may occur. This is an indication of physical, emotional or mental toxins leaving the body, or your environment, and is all part of the body holistically healing itself. It occurs particularly in stress-related or chronic conditions caused by environmental factors or psychic attack. It can be soothed and facilitated by an essence made from crystals such as Smoky Elestial Quartz, Eye of the Storm, Spirit Quartz or Quantum Quattro and by drinking plenty of water (Shungite-infused water is ideal). If a healing challenge occurs, discontinue use for a few days until the symptoms dissipate, then gradually reintroduce the essence you were using – having dowsed or intuited if it is still appropriate.

Part IV

Chakra and auric essences

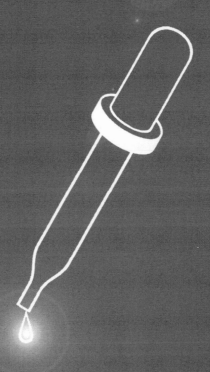

The Chakras

The chakras are multi-layered, multidimensional vortexes of subtle energy that radiate several feet out from your physical body. Linkage points between the physical and subtle energy bodies, they are metaphysical rather than physical but they are essential to our efficient functioning in the world and to raising our consciousness… they act like a vortex or valve, regulating the flow of energy through the subtle and physical bodies via the meridian, endocrine and nervous systems. Chakras mediate how much energy and feelings you take in from the world around you, and your response to that outer world.
– Crystal Prescriptions volume 4

The chakras have an essential part to play in well-being at every level. Each chakra 'governs' an area of life and an organ or part of the body and has to do with specific thoughts and emotions. Stress, tension, distortion or sluggishness in a chakra will ultimately manifest as dis-ease within the physical body or be reflected in psycho-somatic or psychological distress. Restore the equilibrium and rebalance the chakra, and the dis-ease or distress disappears. Crystal essences are ideal for this purpose.

How active your chakras are and whether they are stressed or functioning at optimum powerfully affects your perceptions and your emotions, and how you express your inner world. If they are blocked or overactive, they allow subconscious fears and feelings to rule unchallenged. If they are operating well, they test and challenge perceptions and experiences rather than blindly following the same old pathway. This is why the chakras are so important in human and soul evolution. They assist in assimilating downloads of higher vibrational energy that lift the soul beyond what has been known before.

The chakras range from earthy 'lower' chakras, which vibrate deeply and slowly and ground energy, to 'high vibration' higher chakras that vibrate at a faster, more refined rate and access cosmic consciousness. Mediating between the inner and outer worlds and your physical body and the energies of earth, the earthy chakras assist in assimilating energies and frequencies at the lower level of the scale. They also affect how well or otherwise your body, emotions and mind function. Roughly speaking, the chakras in the belly correspond to the physical level of being, those in the upper torso to the emotional and, from the throat upwards into the skull, the mental level. Chakras above the head work mainly at the spiritual level. They work in conjunction with the subtle auric bodies that are closest in frequency to those levels of being.

[The information in this section has been extracted from *Crystal Prescriptions volume 4* and *Judy Hall's Crystal Companion*.]

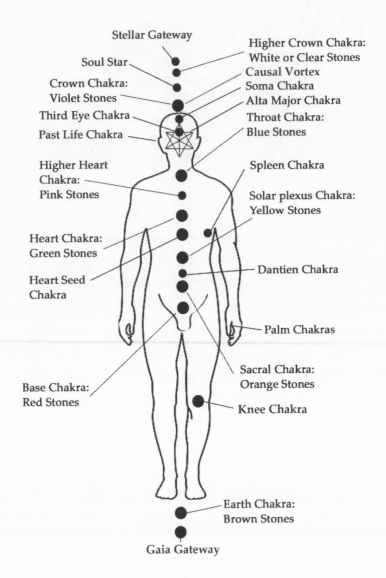

Stellar Gateway

Soul Star

Crown Chakra:
Violet Stones

Third Eye Chakra

Past Life Chakra

Higher Heart
Chakra:
Pink Stones

Heart Chakra:
Green Stones

Heart Seed
Chakra

Base Chakra:
Red Stones

Higher Crown Chakra:
White or Clear Stones
Causal Vortex
Soma Chakra
Alta Major Chakra
Throat Chakra:
Blue Stones

Spleen Chakra

Solar plexus Chakra:
Yellow Stones

Dantien Chakra

Palm Chakras

Sacral Chakra:
Orange Stones

Knee Chakra

Earth Chakra:
Brown Stones

Gaia Gateway

Crystals and the Chakras

Chakra healing

Traditionally, each chakra is linked to specific organs and has its own colour, although, as we will see, there are also other differently coloured crystals that relate to the chakras because the present colour system is a modern one. It is a question of resonance and harmony rather than simply colour. Certain crystals will stimulate a sluggish chakra, others will slow down an overactive one – the A-Z directory has a comprehensive list. If a chakra is spinning too rapidly or is stuck open, using a complementary coloured crystal from the opposite side of the colour wheel (see page 81) could bring it back to equilibrium. Simply select a crystal of a colour from the opposite side of the wheel to the 'traditional' chakra colour, or possibly from the right-angle cross on the colour wheel to harmonise the two ends of the spectrum. Then dowse to check that the essence will work for you – you may need to combine crystals. A crystal of the same traditional colour as the chakra usually stimulates a sluggish or blocked spin. By using crystals of the *appropriate* colour and vibration for chakra essences, chakra imbalances are quickly eliminated and the chakras harmonised to work together, leading to better health and a sense of well-being.

'Traditional' chakra colours

Chakra	Colour
Gaia Gateway	black, brown, silver, gold
Earth Star	brown, dark grey, maroon
Knee	multicoloured, tan
Base	red
Sacral	orange
Dantien	reddish-orange, amber
Solar Plexus	yellow, light greenish yellow
Spleen	green
Heart Seed	pale pearlescent blue, pink, white
Heart	green/pink
Higher Heart	pink, gold, purple, blue
Palm	silver-white, golden-white, red, blue
Throat	blue, turquoise
Third Eye	indigo
Soma	blue, lavender, white, ultraviolet
Crown	white, purple, lavender
Stellar Gateway	deep violet, white, gold, silver or clear
Soul Star	magenta, white, black
Alta Major	magenta, green
Causal Vortex	white, gold

The Colour Wheel

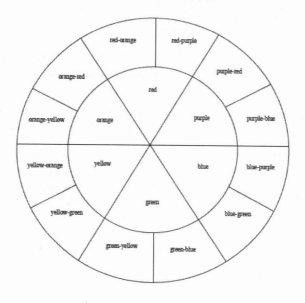

Chakra spin

The chakras whirl and it is not so much the direction of spin that matters but rather the speed *and whether it is an appropriate direction for the individual and the particular chakra*. Each person has a direction of spin that is right for them, which can be checked by dowsing. Occasionally the direction of spin needs to be reversed but more often it is the rate that needs adjusting. Whether a chakra is open or closed affects how energy flows through it, but so too does the speed of rotation. If a chakra is spinning too slowly it will be sluggish and blocked, deficient in energy, so that it cannot mediate flow or receive fresh input. If it is spinning too rapidly then it is stuck open and energy will be whirling in and out without restraint. Crystal essences adjust the rate – and direction – of spin to optimum and assist with opening and closing the chakras as appropriate.

If a chakra is stuck open and spinning too fast, this may be because the chakras above and/or below it have blockages and are stagnant and toxic so that energy cannot circulate freely along the spine and through the subtle bodies. So those chakras would also need treating. The aim is to have all the chakras balanced and functioning at optimum.

Blown or blocked chakra

If a chakra is stuck open and spinning too fast, it is known as a blown chakra. A blown chakra is particularly vulnerable to outside influence as there is no protection or mediation of the energy flow. A blown chakra may be quite literally 'blown away', that is, out of line with the other chakras. If when dowsing or checking how chakra energy is flowing it veers off towards one or other sides of the body, then the chakra will need bringing back into line. That is, it needs to be aligned not only in spin and energetic frequency with the other chakras but also moved back into vertical alignment. An alignment essence will be required.

Similarly, a chakra can be stuck in the closed position – and energy may divert around it. Deficient in energy, a blocked chakra leads to blockages and negative qualities manifesting. A chakra may be blocked because of your own past input, conscious or otherwise, or because other people 'put a block' on it – that is they seek to control you, don't want you to see something, and so on. Chakra blockages have many issues and it pays to search for the deeper cause (see *Crystal Prescriptions volume 4*).

What blocks a chakra?

There are many reasons why a chakra may become blocked or blown and to some extent this depends on where the chakra is situated along the line. Geopathic stress, electromagnetic pollution and too long spent under artificial rather than natural light has a profound effect on the physical body and its associated chakras. But old traumas, toxicity, close-mindedness and fixed beliefs, emotional pain and physical injuries can all contribute. They become an energetic pattern or engram that is imprinted into the appropriate chakra or subtle energy body at a very deep level. Essences from the emotional and mental healing section will be of assistance in this case. However, one of the major causes of blocked or blown chakras is past life issues that have been carried over into the present life. The A-Z karmic and past life healing directory covers crystals to create an essence to remedy a wide range of these past life causes (see page 106). These issues are imprinted in the karmic subtle energy body and the past life and causal vortex chakras so essences dispersed around the aura and head are extremely effective. The layers may need to be peeled back gently over a period of time until the core issue is reached. It can then be released and the energy transmuted.

The Chakras

Gaia Gateway
Planetary soul connection

Location: Deep beneath feet

Function: Connecting your soul to the soul and spirit of Earth, Gaia and Mother Earth, the Gaia gateway assimilates and anchors high vibrations into the physical body and that of Earth adjusting your EMF frequency to remain in harmonic resonance with that of the planet. *Functioning optimally:* You are aware of being a part of a sacred whole. (The Gaia gateway is energetically linked to the stellar gateway.)

Earth Star
Anchoring and grounding

Location: Beneath feet

Function: The earth star is a place of safety and regeneration, keeping you grounded. Connecting to Earth's electromagnetic fields and energy meridians, it goes deep into the core. Actualising plans and dreams, it anchors new frequencies and downloads of cosmic information, creating a stable and strong centre. *Functioning optimally:* Creates a natural electrical circuit and a powerful source of vital energy. (The earth star is energetically linked to the soul star.)

Knees
Flexibility, balance and willpower

Location: Knees

Function: All major energy meridians pass through the knees as does the sciatic nerve, the longest in the body. Knee chakras facilitate nurturing and supporting yourself, manifesting what you need day to day. *Functioning optimally:* You are flexible, able to adapt to changing circumstances, going with the flow yet having perseverance when required. Well balanced knee chakras support in stepping forward into a new way of being.

Base (root)
Basic survival instincts and security issues

Location: Base of spine

Function: Relating to your roots, willpower and ability to make things happen, this is where you connect with your tribe, and where you feel safe. You discover yourself as an individual and take responsibility for your Self. It represents home and career and how secure you feel in each. Imbalances lead to sexual disturbances and 'stuckness', anger, impotence and frustration – and inability to let go. Linking core connection to Earth, the 'sacred bone' is where kundalini rests before it is awakened. *Functioning optimally:* You trust the universe and feel secure.

Sacral
Creativity, passion and fertility

Location: Below navel

Function: An important part of the core energy system, the sacral stimulates production of 'feel good' hormones, having a powerful effect on moment to moment mood. It holds boundaries steady. This is where you handle the immediate environment and matters such as money, career and authority figures. It affects how easily you express your sexuality and how you feel about relationships, holding parenting issues and connection to family in addition to hooks from previous relationships. *Functioning optimally:* You have the ability to bring things into manifestation.

Dantien
Power

Location: Below navel, above sacral
Function: An energy storage vault, when the dantien is full, you have inner resources on which to draw. You are literally power-full. An adjunct to the sacral chakra and point of balance for the physical body, the dantien stores Qi, lifeforce, and earths the body. *Functioning optimally:* A place of inner strength, stability and balance, connected to the dantien, you have more physical energy and are unaffected by life's ups and downs, emotionally stable and able to resist stress.

Navel ('Tummy button')
Nurturing

Location: Centre line, below waist
Function: A potent ancestral line connection point, the

navel links to the mother and matriarchal line. The navel is vulnerable, this is known as the tummy 'button' for good, largely unconscious, reasons as it is the trigger for ancestral memories, especially fear and trauma. Transgenerational messages, DNA, cellular disorders, and matriarchal imperatives lodge here plus ancestral strengths and feminine wisdom. *Functioning optimally:* The soul feels centred in the body, nurtured and grounded. You are able to nurture and accept yourself without relying on external validation. This is where you access the positive qualities of the matriarchal line and pass these on to future generations.

Palms
Energy manifestation, transmutation and utilisation
Location: Palms, fingers, lower arms
Function: Interacting with the world on an energetic level, palms are powerful sensors, where you experience expanded awareness, collecting and radiating energy and impressions. *Functioning optimally:* Palm chakras receive energy from the universe – or crystals – and channel this into another energy field. Palms increase creativity in the physical and subtle energy worlds.

Solar Plexus
Emotions
Location: Above navel
Function: Emotions stored in the solar plexus have a

deeply psychosomatic effect. The point of digestion on all levels, it is where you assimilate nourishment and absorb energy and emotions from outside yourself. Emotional 'hooks' from other people locate here. Having a powerful effect on ability to assert your will, this chakra governs self-confidence and self-esteem in addition to emotional stability. *Functioning optimally:* Linked to intuition, it is the seat of 'gut instincts' and bodily knowing.

Spleen
Self-protection and empowerment
Location: Below left armpit
Function: A seat of power, the spleen is where energy pirates hook in to get their fix, leaving you depleted at immune and vitality levels. *Functioning optimally:* Energy easily flows around the physical and subtle bodies and you are protected.

Heart Seed
Soul remembrance
Location: Tip of breastbone
Function: A soul linkage point, the heart seed recalls the reason for incarnation, showing how to return to the original soulplan if you have deviated. *Functioning optimally:* Assisting in renegotiating past-its-sell-by-date soul purpose, it activates karmic tools to actualise your soul potential.

Heart
Unconditional love and nurturing

Location: Towards base of breastbone

Function: The heart chakra facilitates unselfish self-love and self-worth, rising above egotism. With the higher heart and heart seed, it forms the three-chambered heart chakra. Integrating the whole chakric line, the heart chakra is the core of your being where the physical body and soul meet. Site of bonds made with other people, it governs relationships and interaction with wider worlds. *Functioning optimally:* You 'live from the heart', safe, compassionate and non-judgemental.

Higher Heart (thymus)
Immunity and well-being

Location: Between heart and throat

Function: Governing physical and psychic immune systems, this centre controls how well you protect yourself and has a profound effect on well-being. The first gland to develop, it is a core component of the body *in utero*, governing which genetic potential is switched on, and how much natural immunity you have. Connecting to ancestral DNA and past life patterning in the body, blockages result in a compromised immune system and consequent dis-ease. *Functioning optimally:* You have natural physical and psychic immunity.

Throat
Communication

Location: Centre of throat

Function: This chakra has a surprising amount to do with willpower and choices that arise in life. Mediating contact with the external world, the throat is where you express yourself, including feelings and emotions coming from the heart or solar plexus as well as thoughts. If closed, there is no outlet for these feelings and thoughts, leading to psychosomatic dis-ease. *Functioning optimally:* Opinions and feelings are clearly communicated.

Third Eye (brow)
Intuition and mental connection

Location: Above and between eyebrows

Function: Where inner sight meets outer vision and bonds into intuitive insight, the third eye sees beyond everyday reality into what really *is*: sensing unseen worlds and higher dimensions. Imbalances result in being bombarded by other people's thoughts, or overwhelmed by irrational intuitions with no basis in truth. Controlling or coercing mental 'hooks' from outside influences lock in here. *Functioning optimally:* Intuition can be relied upon.

Soma
Soulbody connection

Location: Mid hairline above third eye

Function: Where soul and etheric bodies attach to the physical, the soma anchors the 'silver cord' holding subtle energy bodies in contact with the physical. It links to angelic realms and spirit guides. Out of balance, it is easy for the soul to disconnect, or for discarnate spirits to attach, and involuntary out-of-body experiences to occur that may literally blow your mind. *Functioning optimally:* It gives the clarity necessary to achieve en-lighten-ment. Cosmic light anchors the Soulbody to the physical and the greater whole.

Past Life
Memory and hereditary issues

Location: Behind ears

Function: Where memories of previous incarnations are stored together with deeply ingrained soul programs and emotional baggage, past life chakras hold soul contracts, intentions, traumas, dramas, gifts and lessons from many lifetimes. They link to the karmic etheric body that stores soul wounds, physical or emotional, recreating psychosomatic dis-ease or physical disease through subtle DNA memory traces. Activating these chakras brings up memories for release. Soul contracts can resemble curses or hexing moving down a family or karmic line. *Functioning optimally:* Facilitate moving forward with no baggage, freed from karmic deficits, drawing on karmic credits.

Crown
Spiritual communication and awareness

Location: Top of head

Function: A place of spiritual, intellectual and intuitive *knowing*, the crown chakra connects to multidimensions and multiverses. When blocked, excessive environmental sensitivity, delusions or dementia result. *Functioning optimally:* Soul purpose is actualised, leading to self-understanding. Certain of your pathway, you are attuned to the cycles of life, recognising lessons programmed in before birth and soul gifts you seek.

Alta Major (Ascension)
Expanding awareness

Location: Inside and around skull

Function: Anchoring the multidimensional lightbody, the alta major shows the bigger picture. Holding the ancestral past and ingrained patterns that govern human life, in conjunction with the causal vortex and past life chakras, it accesses past life karma and contractual agreements plus the soul's plan. *Functioning optimally:* The subtle endocrine system harmonises auric bodies with the physical. There is a strong sense of direction.

Soul Star
Ultimate soul awareness

Location: Above head

Function: An interface between spirit and matter, out of balance this chakra creates spiritual arrogance, soul fragmentation or a messiah-complex, or is the site of spirit attachment, ET invasion, or overwhelm by ancestral spirits. *Functioning optimally:* This energy centre recalibrates extremely high spiritual frequencies to be assimilated and integrated into matter. (The soul star is energetically linked to the earth star.)

Stellar Gateway
Cosmic doorway to other worlds

Location: Above soul star

Function: A dimensional portal, the stellar gateway connects to the divine and to multiverses. When this chakra is imbalanced, the soul is a 'space cadet', fragmented, disintegrated, unable to function in the everyday world. *Functioning optimally:* Two-way communication with higher dimensional beings is facilitated and spiritual illumination results. (The stellar gateway is energetically linked to the Gaia gateway.)

Causal Vortex
Soul journey

Location: Above and to side of head

Function: A universal and cosmic worldswide web, the causal vortex accesses the Akashic Records to reveal how far you've travelled on your spiritual journey. A repository for ancestral and karmic dis-eases, it brings subtle and physical bodies into alignment, activating DNA potential. *Functioning optimally:* Wisdom and guidance illuminating lessons planned and highlighting karmic skills and abilities is received and integrated.

The Chakras and Physiology

The chakras link to energy management, specific organs and the endocrine system.

Gaia Gateway
Physiology: Subtle energy bodies, linking into Earth's subtle bodies and meridian system. *Typical dis-eases:* Supra-physical. Inability to ground kundalini and higher frequencies leads to subtle dis-ease.

Earth Star
Physiology: Physical body, electrical and meridian systems, sciatic nerve, sensory organs. *Typical dis-eases:* Lethargic or invasive. M.E., arthritis, cancer, muscular disorders, depression, psychiatric disturbances, autoimmune diseases, persistent tiredness.

Knee
Physiology: Brain, kidneys, lumbar spine, heart, bladder and kidney meridians, sciatic nerve. *Typical dis-eases:* Disabling. Knee problems, arthritis, cartilage and joint problems, bladder infections, cold feet, Raynaud's Disease, Osgood-Schlatter syndrome, bursitis, osteoarthritis, poor leg circulation, sacroiliac pain, eating disorders, malabsorption of nutrients, kidney diseases.

Palm
Physiology: Nerves, tendons, ganglions, skin, hands,

fingers, nails. *Typical dis-eases:* Incapacitating. Arthritis, brittle nails, carpal tunnel, Dupytren's contracture, eczema, plantar fasciitis, psoriasis, rashes, allergies, shin splints, gut-disturbances, repetitive strain injury.

Base

Physiology: 'Fight or flight' response, adrenals, bladder, elimination and immune systems, gonads, kidneys, lower back, lower extremities, sciatic nerve, lymph system, prostate gland, rectum, teeth and bones, veins. *Typical dis-eases:* Constant, low level, or flare up. Adrenal response is permanently activated. Stiffness or tingling in joints, poor circulation in lower limbs, sciatica, chronic lower back pain; renal, reproductive or rectal disorders; fluid retention, constipation or diarrhoea, prostate problems, haemorrhoids, varicose veins or hernias, bipolar disorder, addictions, glandular disturbances, personality and anxiety disorders, skeletal/bone/teeth problems, autoimmune diseases; insomnia and disturbed sleep, waking unrefreshed.

Sacral

Physiology: Bladder and gallbladder, immune and elimination systems, kidneys, large and small intestine, lumbar and pelvic region, sacrum, spleen, ovaries, testes, uterus. *Typical dis-eases:* Pernicious and psychosomatic. PMT, muscle cramps, sciatica, reproductive blockages or diseases, prostate problems, impotence, infertility, fibroids, endometriosis, allergies, addictions, eating disorders, diabetes, liver or intestinal dysfunction, irritable bowel syndrome, chronic back pain, urinary infections.

Dantien

Physiology: Autonomic nervous and energy-conduction systems, regulation of internal organs and involuntary processes such as breathing and heartbeat. Sensory impulses to the brain. *Typical dis-eases:* Physical dysfunction. Nervous system disturbance, autoimmune diseases, cardiac problems, high blood pressure, orthostatic hypotension, palpitations, adrenal overload, chronic fatigue, M.E., Raynaud's, Parkinson's Disease, digestive problems, diabetes, lightheadedness, powerlessness, ill at ease in incarnation.

Navel

Physiology: DNA, RNA and 'junk DNA', epigenetics, blood and lymphatic system, uterus and reproductive area, autonomic nervous system, filtration systems. *Typical dis-eases:* Inherited through the matriarchal line. Difficulty in giving birth. Deeply ingrained fears trigger autoimmune diseases and endocrine malfunctions. If the mother's womb was noxious and toxic, breathing difficulties result.

Solar Plexus

Physiology: Adrenals, digestive system, liver, lymphatic system, metabolism, muscles, pancreas, skin, small intestine, stomach, eyesight. *Typical dis-eases:* Emotional and demanding. Stomach ulcers, M.E., adrenaline imbalances, S.A.D. (seasonal affective disorder), insomnia and chronic anxiety, digestive problems, malabsorption of nutrients, gallstones, pancreatic failure, liver problems, eczema and skin conditions, eating disorders, phobias, multiple sclerosis.

Heart Seed

Physiology: Integrated physical and subtle energy systems. *Typical dis-eases:* Depletion and disillusionment at a spiritual level.

Heart

Physiology: Chest, circulation, heart, lungs, shoulders, thymus, respiratory system. *Typical dis-eases:* Psychosomatic and reactive. Heart attacks, angina, chest infections, asthma, frozen shoulder, ulcers, persistent cough, wheeziness, pneumonia, high cholesterol, mastitis, breast cysts, pancreatic problems.

Higher Heart (thymus)

Physiology: Psychic and physical immune systems, thymus gland, lymphatic system, elimination and purification organs. *Typical dis-eases:* Disordered immune system. Autoimmune diseases, repeated viral and bacterial infections, coughs, colds, glandular fever, M.E., M.S., HIV/Aids, arteriosclerosis, flushing of chest and neck, tinnitus, epilepsy, vitiligo, psoriasis, alopecia, thyroid problems.

Spleen

Physiology: Spleen, pancreas, lymphatic system and liver. *Typical dis-eases:* Depletion and lack. Lethargy, anaemia, low blood sugar, diabetes, pancreatitis, liver problems, autoimmune diseases.

Throat

Physiology: Ears, nose, respiratory and nervous system, sinuses, skin, throat, thyroid, parathyroid, tongue, tonsils, speech and body language, metabolism. *Typical dis-eases:* Block communication. Sore throat/quinsy, lump in throat, difficulty in swallowing, inflammation of trachea, sinus, constant colds and viral infections, tinnitus, ear infections, jaw pain, gum disease, tooth problems, thyroid imbalances, high blood pressure, ADHD, autism, speech impediment, irritable bowel, psychosomatic and metabolic dis-eases.

Third Eye (brow)

Physiology: Brain, ears, eyes, neurological and endocrine systems, pineal and pituitary glands, hypothalamus, production of serotonin and melatonin, temperature control, scalp, sinuses. *Typical dis-eases:* Metaphysical. Migraine, mental overwhelm, schizophrenia, cataracts, iritis, epilepsy, autism, spinal and neurological disorders, sinus and ear infections, high blood pressure, learning disabilities, memory loss, eye problems. Nervous or hormonal disorders, hot or cold flushes, excessive perspiration, 'irritations'; skin conditions such as psoriasis, eczema, impetigo, hives; allergies, sinus problems, adenoid and ear disorders, lack of energy and/or sex drive.

Soma

Physiology: Whole body including etheric bodies, subtle energy systems and meridians, pineal and pituitary glands. *Typical dis-eases:* Autistic, disconnected, dyspraxic. Down's Syndrome, autism, ADHD, chronic fatigue, delusional states, sinus or eye problems, migraine headaches, stress headaches, digestive difficulties.

Past Life

Physiology: Karmic blueprint and etheric bodies. Wounds, attitudes and dysfunction in subtle bodies imprint on to the physical at a psychosomatic or genetic level. Psychological dis-eases impact on mind and body. *Typical dis-eases:* Chronic. Immune or endocrine deficiencies, genetic or physical malfunctions; heart, liver or kidney problems; autoimmune diseases.

Crown

Physiology: Brain, central nervous system, hair, hypothalamus, pituitary gland, spine, subtle energy bodies, cerebellum, nervous and motor control, posture and balance. *Typical dis-eases:* Disconnection and isolation. Metabolic syndrome, hypertension, 'vague unwellness', lethargy, nervous system disturbances, electromagnetic and environmental sensitivity, depression, dementia, M.E., Parkinson's Disease, insomnia or excessive sleepiness, 'biological clock' disturbances, seasonal affective disorder (S.A.D.), impaired coordination, headaches, migraine, anxiety, insomnia, depression, multiple personality disorder, mental breakdown.

Alta Major

Physiology: Subtle and physical endocrine systems, hippocampus, hypothalamus, pineal and pituitary glands; brain function, cerebellum, voluntary muscle movements, medulla oblongata, breathing, heart rate and blood pressure; hormonal balance, occipital area and optic nerves, throat, spine, sleeping patterns. *Typical dis-eases:* Inherited and karmic. Disorientation, metabolic dysfunction, eye problems, floaters, cataracts, migraine, headaches, memory loss, Alzheimer's or dementia, confusion, physical depression, 'dizziness' or disconnection, loss of purpose, spiritual depression, fear, terror, adrenaline rush.

Soul Star

Physiology: Subtle bodies and the psyche. *Typical dis-eases:* Psychological and psychiatric. Schizophrenia, paranoia, bipolar disorder.

Stellar Gateway

Physiology: Beyond physical. *Typical dis-eases:* Spiritual and soul disconnection.

Causal Vortex

Physiology: Etheric and karmic blueprint, inherited and karmic diseases, DNA and RNA. *Typical dis-eases:* Ancestral and karmic.

For further information on the chakras, see Crystal Prescriptions volume 4.

Auric and subtle bodies

Biomagnetic fields, subtle energy bodies radiate out from the physical body in interpenetrating waves, connecting via the chakras. These auric fields link to multidimensional frequencies and are blueprints holding information, bio-memories and engrams from which the physical body is constructed. Crystal essences entrain the subtle bodies back into equilibrium, healing energetic 'holes', energy depletion, distortion or imprinted patterns that no longer serve and which, ultimately, create physical dis-ease.

Physical-etheric body

Function: A biomagnetic program holding imprints of past life dis-ease, injuries and beliefs, the physical-etheric body contains subtle DNA activated or switched off by behaviour, emotions and beliefs. This in turn affects DNA in the physical body.

Chakra connection: Seven traditional, lower frequency chakras and soma, past life, alta major and causal vortex chakras.

Emotional body

Function: Imprinted with emotions and feelings, attitudes, heartbreaks, traumas and dramas from present and previous lives, the emotional body contains engrams, bundles of energy holding deeply traumatic or joyful memory pictures. Dis-ease in this body is reflected in the knees and feet, which act out insecurities and fears, or heart and abdomen.

Chakra connection: Knees, solar plexus, base and sacral, throat, heart.

Mental body

Function: Created from thoughts, memories, credos and ingrained limiting beliefs from past and present lives, the mental body holds imprints of authority figures from the past, along with inculcated ideologies, attitudes and points of view.

Chakra connection: Throat and head chakras and lower body.

Karmic body

Function: Holding imprints of all previous lives and the purpose for the present life, the karmic body contains mental programs, physical imprints, emotional impressions and beliefs that may be contradictory and create internal conflict. When balanced, evolutionary intent is actualised.

Chakra connection: Past life, alta major and causal vortex chakras may affect soma, knee and earth star.

Ancestral body

Function: Everything that is inherited down both sides of ancestral lineage at the physical, or more subtle, levels is held in the ancestral body including family sagas, belief systems, attitudes, culture, loss, expectations, traumas and dramas. Healing sent down the ancestral line to the core experience rebounds forward to heal the future. Ancestral imperatives must be released before soul evolution occurs.

Chakra connection: Soul star, past life, alta major, causal vortex, higher heart, earth star and Gaia gateway chakras.

Planetary body

Function: Linking into the physical planet and Earth's etheric body and meridians, the planetary body connects to the wider cosmos, luminaries, planets and stellar bodies. Cosmic or soul dis-ease is corrected through the planetary subtle body.

Chakra connection: Past life, alta major, causal vortex, soma, stellar and Gaia gateway chakras.

Spiritual or Lightbody

Function: An integrated, luminous, vibrating energy field, the lightbody connects the physical body, subtle energy bodies, with spirit or soul and the wider cosmos.

Chakra connection: All especially soma, soul star, stellar gateway, Gaia gateway, alta major and causal vortex.

A-Z Directory of chakra and auric essences

Choose 1–4 crystals from an entry when creating your essence.

– A –

Activate all chakras: Anandalite™, Brookite, Fulgarite, Golden Healer Quartz, Green Ridge Quartz, Phlogopite, Rhodozite, Triplite, Victorite *and see Chakras page 76 and individual chakra entries*

Align:

all chakras, especially third eye and crown or higher crown to the lightbody through the soul star: Anandalite™, Vera Cruz Amethyst

balance and activate base through to heart chakras: Bloodstone, Carnelian, Green Ridge Quartz, Triplite

lightbody to the physical body through the lower chakra system and to the divine through the higher vibration chakras: Golden Coracalcite

mind-body-spirit: Aurichalcite, Eye of the Storm, Golden Coracalcite, Green Ridge Quartz, Lavikite, Sillimanite. *Chakra:* alta major (base of skull) and dantien

physical and subtle bodies: Alexandrite, Anandalite™, Aurichalcite, Empowerite, Fulgarite, Golden Coracalcite, Golden Healer, Green Ridge Quartz, Herderite, Lemurian Seed, Mount Shasta Opal, Nuummite, Paraiba Tourmaline, Schalenblende,

Scheelite, Sillimanite, Thompsonite, Zincite. *Chakra:* alta major (base of skull), soma

the chakras: Afghanite, Amber, Anandalite™, Annabergite, Barite, Black Kyanite, Chrysoprase, Citrine, Gaia Stone, Kyanite, Lemurian Seed, Lepidocrosite, Paraiba Tourmaline, Picrolite, Pink Kunzite, Quartz, Shungite, Sichuan Quartz, Sillimanite, Sodalite

> **Align physical with multidimensional consciousness:** Citrine
> **Align with etheric bodies:** Anandalite
> **Align with lightbody:** Anandalite, Green Ridge Quartz
> **Align with physical body:** Amber, Anandalite, Shungite

Alta major chakra: Afghanite, African Jade (Budd Stone), Anandalite, Andara Glass, Angelinite, Angel's Wing Calcite, Apatite, Auralite 23, Aurichalcite, Azeztulite, Black Moonstone, Blue Moonstone, Brandenberg Amethyst, Crystal Cap Amethyst, Diaspore (Zultanite), Emerald, Ethiopian Opal, Eye of the Storm (Judy's Jasper), Fire and Ice Quartz, Fluorapatite, Garnet in Pyroxene, Graphic Smoky Quartz, Green Ridge Quartz, Golden Healer, Golden Herkimer Diamond, Holly Agate, Hungarian Quartz, Petalite, Phenacite, Preseli Bluestone, Rainbow Covellite, Rainbow Mayanite, Red Agate, Red Amethyst, Rosophia. *Disperse at base of skull.*

> **balance and align:** Anandalite, Brandenberg

Amethyst, Crystal Cap Amethyst, Green Ridge Quartz, Preseli Bluestone. Rub gently on soma chakra with Angel's Wing Calcite or Herkimer Diamond.

spin too rapid/stuck open: African Jade (Budd Stone), Auralite 23, Black Moonstone, Calcite, Eye of the Storm, Flint, Golden Healer, Graphic Smoky Quartz

spin too sluggish/stuck closed: Blue Moonstone, Diaspore, Ethiopian Opal, Herkimer Diamond, Quartz, Red Agate

Ancestral body: Anthrophyllite, Blue Holly Agate, Brandenberg Amethyst, Bumble Bee Jasper, Candle Quartz, Catlinite, Datolite, Eclipse Stone, Fairy Quartz, Icicle Calcite, Ilmenite, Jade, Kambaba Jasper, Lemurian Aquatine Calcite, Mohawkite, Peanut Wood, Petrified Wood, Porphyrite, Prasiolite, Rainbow Mayanite, Rainforest Jasper, Shaman Quartz, Smoky Elestial Quartz, Spirit Quartz, Starseed, Stromatolite. *Chakra:* soul star, past life, alta major, causal vortex, higher heart, earth star and Gaia gateway

Aura: Anandalite™, Beryllonite, Quartz, Scolecite

align with physical body: Ajo Blue Calcite, Amber, Anandalite, Candle Quartz, Empowerite, Fulgarite, Lavikite, Orange Sphalerite, Schalenblende, Scheelite, Scolecite, Sichuan Quartz, Sillimanite, Thompsonite

blockages, remove: Ajo Quartz, Anandalite, Arfvedsonite, Beryllonite, Charoite, Fire and Ice Quartz, Flint, Fulgarite, Jasper, Prehnite with Epidote, Rainbow Mayanite, Rhodozite, Serpentine in Obsidian

cleansing: Amber, Amechlorite, Anandalite, Black Kyanite, Bloodstone, Citrine Spirit Quartz, Fire and Ice Quartz, Flint, Fulgarite, Green Jasper, Herkimer Diamond, Holly Agate, Keyiapo, Lepidocrosite, Mystic Topaz, Nuummite, Phlogopite, Pumice, Pyrite in Quartz, Pyrite and Sphalerite, Quartz, Rainbow Mayanite, Rutile, Smoky Quartz. 'Comb' aura thoroughly.

energize: Anandalite™, Gold in Quartz, Iolite, Quartz, Rainbow Mayanite, Sichuan Quartz, Triplite. *Chakra:* solar plexus

energy leakage, guard against: Eudialyte, Gaspeite, Healer's Gold, Labradorite, Pyrite in Quartz, Quartz with Mica, Spectrolite. *Chakra:* higher heart. *Disperse or spritz around aura.*

heal: Anandalite, Keyiapo, Scolecite, Sichuan Quartz, Smoky Amethyst, Tugtupite

'holes'/breaks: Aegerine, Amethyst, Aqua Aura, Brookite, Chinese Red Quartz, Eye of the Storm, Flint, Green Ridge Quartz, Green Tourmaline, Labradorite, Lemurian Seed, Quartz, Scolecite, Selenite. *Disperse over site.*

negativity, remove: Amber, Apache Tear, Black Jade, Fulgarite, Nuummite with Novaculite, Smoky Amethyst, Spectrolite, Tantalite. *Chakra:* solar plexus

protect: Amber, Amethyst, Apache Tear, Brandenberg Amethyst, Diamond, Hackmanite, Honey Phantom Calcite, Labradorite, Mahogany Sheen Obsidian, Master Shamanite, Nunderite, Orgonite, Paraiba

Tourmaline, Quartz, Shattuckite with Ajoite, Tantalite. *Chakra:* higher heart. *Disperse around aura.*

repattern: Anandalite, Brandenberg Amethyst, Cradle of Life (Humanity), Golden Lemurian Seed, Iolite-and-Sunstone, Lapis Lace, Rainbow Lattice Sunstone, Rainbow Mayanite, Sea Foam Flint, Strawberry Lemurian Seed

seal: Actinolite, Andean Blue Opal, Brookite, Feather Pyrite, Fulgarite, Galaxyite, Healer's Gold, Honey Phantom Calcite, Labradorite, Lorenzite (Ramsayite), Molybdenite in Quartz, Nunderite, Pyromorphite, Serpentine in Obsidian, Smoky Amethyst, Spectrolite, Tantalite, Thunder Egg, Valentinite and Stibnite, Xenotine

stabilise: Agate, Fulgarite, Granite, Labradorite, Mtrolite, Poppy Jasper. *Chakra:* earth star

strengthen: Ajo Blue Calcite, Anandalite, Brookite, Ethiopian Opal, Flint, Magnetite (Lodestone), Quartz Tantalite, Thunder Egg, Zircon

– B –

Base chakra: Amber, Azurite, Bastnasite, Black Obsidian, Black Opal, Black Tourmaline, Bloodstone, Candle Quartz, Carnelian, Chinese Red Quartz, Chrysocolla, Cinnabar Jasper, Citrine, Clinohumite, Cuprite, Dragon Stone, Eye of the Storm (Judy's Jasper), Fire Agate, Fulgarite, Gabbro, Garnet, Golden Topaz, Harlequin Quartz (Hematite in Quartz), Hematite, Kambaba Jasper, Keyiapo, Limonite, Obsidian, Pink Tourmaline, Poppy

Jasper, Realgar and Orpiment, Red Amethyst, Red Calcite, Red Jasper, Red Zincite, Ruby, Serpentine, Serpentine in Obsidian, Shungite, Smoky Quartz, Sonora Sunrise, Spinel, Stromatolite, Tangerose, Triplite, Zircon

balance and align: Anandalite, Celestobarite, Green Ridge Quartz, Hematite Quartz, Red Calcite, Red Coral, Ruby, Shiva Lingam

spin too rapid/stuck open: Agate, Green Ridge Quartz, Mahogany Obsidian, Pink Tourmaline, Smoky Quartz, Triplite in matrix

spin too sluggish/stuck closed: Fire Agate, Hematite, Kundalini Quartz, Red Calcite, Serpentine, Sonora Sunrise, Triplite

– C –

Causal vortex chakra: Ajoite, Apatite, Azeztulite, Banded White Agate, Black or Blue Moonstone, Blue Kyanite, Brandenberg Amethyst, Chrysotile, Cobalto Calcite, Cryolite, Crystalline Blue Kyanite, Diamond, Diaspore (Zultanite), Fluorapatite, Herderite, Petalite, Phenacite, Rainbow Moonstone, Scolecite, Sugilite, Tanzanite

balance and align: Anandalite, Brandenberg Amethyst, Chrysotile, Crystalline Blue Kyanite, Fluorapatite, Phenacite, Scolecite, Smoky Elestial Quartz

spin too rapid/stuck open: Black Moonstone, Cobalto Calcite, Diaspore, Scolecite with Natrolite

spin too sluggish/stuck closed: Ajoite, Blue

Moonstone, Herderite, Petalite, Tanzanite

Crown chakra: Afghanite, Amethyst, Amphibole Quartz, Angelite, Angel's Wing Calcite, Arfvedsonite, Auralite 23, Brandenberg Amethyst, Brookite, Celestial Quartz, Citrine, Clear Tourmaline, Diaspore (Zultanite), Golden Beryl, Golden Healer, Green Ridge Quartz, Herderite, Heulandite, Larimar, Lepidolite, Moldavite, Natrolite, Novaculite, Petalite, Phenacite, Purple Jasper, Purple Sapphire, Quartz, Rosophia, Satyamani and Satyaloka Quartz, Scolecite, Selenite, Serpentine, Sugilite, Titanite (Sphene), Trigonic, White Calcite, White Topaz

> **balance and align:** Amethyst, Anandalite, Auralite 23, Brandenberg Amethyst, Phenacite, Selenite, Sugilite
>
> **spin too rapid/stuck open:** Amethyst, Amphibole Quartz, Larimar, Petalite, Serpentine, White Calcite
>
> **spin too sluggish/stuck closed:** Moldavite, Phenacite, Rosophia, Selenite

– D –

Dantien chakra: Amber, Carnelian, Chinese Red Quartz, Empowerite, Eye of the Storm, Fire Agate, Fire Opal, Golden Herkimer, Green Ridge Quartz, Hematite, Hematoid Calcite, Kambaba Jasper, Madagascan Red 'Celestial Quartz', Moonstone, Orange River Quartz, Peanut Wood, Polychrome Jasper, Poppy Jasper, Red Amethyst, Red Jasper, Rhodozite, Rose or Ruby Aura Quartz, Rosophia, Stromatolite, Topaz

> **balance and align:** Empowerite, Eye of the Storm, Green Ridge Quartz, Poppy Jasper

spin too rapid/stuck open: Peanut Wood, Polychrome Jasper, Stromatolite

spin too sluggish/stuck closed: Fire Agate, Fire Opal, Hematite, Madagascan Red 'Celestial Quartz', Poppy Jasper, Red Jasper

– E –

Earth star chakra: Agnitite™, Boji Stone, Brown Jasper, Celestobarite, Champagne Aura Quartz, Cuprite, Fire Agate, Flint, Galena (wash hands after use, create essence by indirect method), Golden Herkimer, Graphic Smoky Quartz, Hematite, Lemurian Jade, Limonite, Madagascan Red 'Celestial Quartz', Mahogany Obsidian, Proustite, Red Amethyst, Rhodonite, Rhodozite, Rosophia, Smoky Elestial Quartz, Smoky Quartz, Thunder Egg, Tourmaline

balance and align: Blue Flint, Brown-flash Anandalite, Green Ridge Quartz, Hematite, Smoky Elestial Quartz

spin too rapid/stuck open: Flint, Graphic Smoky Quartz, Green Ridge Quartz, Smoky Quartz

spin too sluggish/stuck closed: Golden Herkimer, Hematite, Red Amethyst, Rhodozite, Thunder Egg

Emotional body: Apache Tear, Black Moonstone, Blue Moonstone, Botswana (Banded) Agate, Brandenberg Amethyst, Calcite, Danburite, Icicle Calcite, Kunzite, Lepidolite, Mangano Calcite, Moonstone, Pink Moonstone, Pink Petalite, Rainbow Mayanite, Rainbow Moonstone, Rainbow Obsidian, Rhodochrosite,

Rhodonite, Rose Elestial Quartz, Rose Quartz, Rubellite, Selenite, Tourmalinated Quartz, Tugtupite, Watermelon Tourmaline. *Chakra:* solar plexus, three-chambered heart, sacral and base chakras, knees and feet

Etheric body: Andescine Labradorite, Angelinite, Astraline, Brandenberg Amethyst, Chlorite Quartz, Chrysotile, Datolite, Elestial Quartz, Ethiopian Opal, Eye of the Storm, Flint, Girasol, Icicle Calcite, Keyiapo, Khutnohorite, Lemurian Aquitane Calcite, Poldarvarite, Pollucite, Quantum Quattro, Que Sera, Rainbow Mayanite, Rhodozite, Ruby Lavender Quartz, Sanda Rosa Azeztulite, Scheelite, Selenite, Shaman Quartz, Shungite, Stellar Beam Calcite, Tangerine Dream Lemurian, Tantalite. *Chakra:* 7 traditional chakras, plus soma, past life, alta major, causal vortex

– G –

Gaia gateway chakra: Apache Tear, Basalt, Basanite, Black Actinolite, Black Calcite, Black Flint, Black Kyanite, Black Obsidian, Black Petalite, Black Spinel, Black Spot Herkimer Diamond, Day and Night Quartz, Fire and Ice, Jet, Master Shamanite, Mohawkite, Morion, Naturally Dark Smoky Quartz (not irradiated), Nebula Stone, Nirvana Quartz, Nuummite, Petalite, Preseli Bluestone, Sardonyx, Shungite, Smoky Elestial Quartz, Snowflake Obsidian, Specular Hematite, Spiders Web Obsidian, Stromatolite, Tektite, Tibetan Black Spot Quartz, Tourmalinated Quartz, Verdellite

 balance and align: Black Flint, Day and Night Quartz,

Fire and Ice, Master Shamanite, Morion, Shungite, Tourmalinated Quartz, Verdellite

spin too rapid/stuck open: Apache Tear, Basalt, Black Flint, Black Kyanite, Master Shamanite, Sardonyx, Shungite

spin too sluggish/stuck closed: Black Spot Herkimer Diamond, Nirvana Quartz, Preseli Bluestone, Shungite, Specular Hematite, Tektite, Tibetan Black Spot Quartz

– H –

Heart chakra: Apophyllite, Aventurine, Chrysocolla, Chrysoprase, Cobalto Calcite, Danburite, Eudialyte, Gaia Stone, Green Jasper, Green Quartz, Green Sapphire, Green Siberian Quartz, Green Tourmaline, Hematite Quartz, Herkimer Diamond, Jade, Jadeite, Kunzite, Lavender Quartz, Lepidolite, Malachite, Morganite, Muscovite, Pink Danburite, Pink Petalite, Pink Tourmaline, Pyroxmangite, Red Calcite, Rhodochrosite, Rhodonite, Rhodozaz, Rose Quartz, Rubellite Tourmaline, Ruby, Ruby Lavender Quartz, Tugtupite, Variscite, Watermelon Tourmaline

  balance and align: Anandalite, Cobalto Calcite, Kunzite, Mangano Calcite, Ruby Lavender Quartz, Watermelon Tourmaline

  clear heart chakra attachments: Banded Agate, Mangano Calcite

  open the three-chambered heart: Danburite, Lemurian Aquitane Calcite, Mangano Calcite, Pink

Petalite, Pink Tourmaline, Rosophia, Tugtupite

spin too rapid/stuck open: Green Tourmaline, Mangano Calcite, Quartz, Rose Quartz, Tugtupite

spin too sluggish/stuck closed: Calcite, Chohua Jasper, Danburite, Erythrite, Honey Calcite, Lemurian Jade, Pink Lemurian Seed, Red Calcite, Rhodozaz, Rose Quartz, Strawberry Quartz, Tugtupite

Heart seed chakra: Ajo Blue Calcite, Ajoite, Azeztulite, Brandenberg Amethyst, Coral», Danburite, Dianite, Fire Opal, Golden Healer, Green Ridge Quartz, Khutnohorite, Lemurian Calcite, Lilac Quartz, Macedonian Opal, Mangano Calcite, Merkabite Calcite, Pink Opal, Pyroxmangite, Rhodozaz, Roselite, Rosophia, Ruby Lavender Quartz, Scolecite, Spirit Quartz, Tugtupite, Violane

balance and align: Danburite, Golden Healer, Golden Herkimer, Khutnohorite, Merkabite Calcite

spin too rapid/stuck open: Ajo Blue Calcite, Khutnohorite, Macedonian Opal

spin too sluggish/stuck closed: Fire Opal, Rhodozaz, Rosophia, Spirit Quartz

Higher heart chakra: Ajo Blue Calcite, Amazonite, Anandalite (Aurora Quartz), Aqua Aura Quartz, Azeztulite, Bloodstone, Celestite, Danburite, Dioptase, Dream Quartz, Eye of the Storm, Fire and Ice Quartz, Gaia Stone, Green Siberian Quartz, Khutnohorite, Kunzite, Lavender Quartz, Lazurine, Lilac Quartz, Macedonian Opal, Mangano Calcite, Muscovite, Nirvana Quartz, Phenacite, Pink Crackle Quartz, Pink Lazurine,

Pink or Lilac Danburite, Pink Petalite, Pyroxmangite, Quantum Quattro, Que Sera, Rainbow Mayanite, Raspberry Aura Quartz, Rhodozaz, Rose Elestial Quartz, Rose Opal, Rose Quartz, Roselite, Rosophia, Ruby Aura Quartz, Ruby Lavender Quartz™, Spirit Quartz, Strawberry Lemurian, Strawberry Quartz, Tangerose, Tugtupite, Turquoise

> **balance and align:** Bloodstone, Eye of the Storm, Quantum Quattro, Que Sera, Tangerose
>
> **spin too rapid/stuck open:** Eye of the Storm, Mangano Calcite, Pink Petalite, Rose Elestial Quartz, Turquoise
>
> **spin too sluggish/stuck closed:** Quantum Quattro, Que Sera, Ruby Aura Quartz, Strawberry Lemurian

– K –

Karmic body/karmic blueprint: Ammolite, Ammonite, Brandenberg Amethyst, Chrysotile, Cloudy Quartz, Crinoidal Limestone, Datolite, Dumortierite, Flint, Kambaba Jasper, Keyiapo, Khutnohorite, Lemurian Seed, Nirvana Quartz, Rainbow Mayanite, Rhodozite, Ruby Lavender Quartz, Sanda Rosa Azeztulite, Scheelite, Shaman Quartz, Shungite, Stromatolite, Titanite (Sphene) *and see page 242. Chakra:* past life, alta major, causal vortex, soma, knee and earth star

Knee chakras: Aragonite, Azurite, Blue Lace Agate, Boji Stone, Cathedral Quartz, Dinosaur Bone, Flint, Hematite, Magnetite, Merlinite, Peanut Wood, Petrified Wood, Preseli Bluestone, Shungite with Selenite, Sodalite,

Spiders Web Obsidian, Stromatolite

balance and align: Aragonite, Magnetite, Mohawkite, Polychrome Jasper, Preseli Bluestone with chalk

spin too rapid/stuck open: Flint, Hematite, Mohawkite, Polychrome Jasper, Smoky Quartz

spin too sluggish/stuck closed: Fire Opal, Harlequin Quartz, Hematite Quartz

– L –

Lightbody: Agnitite™, Anandalite™, Angel's Wing Calcite, Blue Moonstone, Brandenberg Amethyst, Chlorite Brandenberg, Eklogite, Erythrite, Golden Coracalcite, Golden Healer Quartz, Golden Himalayan Azeztulite, Hackmanite, Himalayan Gold Azeztulite™, Lemurian Seed, Lilac-purple Coquimbite, Madagascan Red 'Celestial Quartz', Mahogany Sheen Obsidian, Merkabite Calcite, Natrolite, Nirvana Quartz, Opal Aura Quartz, Phantom Calcite, Phenacite, Pink Lemurian, Prophecy Stone, Rainbow Mayanite, Red Amethyst, Rutilated Quartz (Angel Hair), Rutile with Hematite, Satyaloka Quartz, Satyamani Quartz, Scolecite, Spirit Quartz, Sugar Blade Quartz, Tangerine Dream Lemurian, Tiffany Stone, Trigonic Quartz, Tugtupite, Vera Cruz Amethyst, Violet Ussingite. *Chakra:* soma, soul star, stellar gateway, Gaia gateway, alta major, causal vortex

– M –

Mental body: Amechlorite, Amethyst, Arfvedsonite, Auralite 23, Brandenberg Amethyst, Celadonite, Chlorite

Brandenberg, Crystal Cap Amethyst, Dumortierite, Fluorite, Lemurian Seed, Merkabite Calcite, Nuummite, Owyhee Blue Opal, Rainbow Covellite, Rainbow Mayanite, Sapphire, Scheelite, Scolecite, Sodalite, Sugilite, Vera Cruz Amethyst. *Chakra:* third eye, soma, alta major, causal vortex

– P –

Palm chakras: Flint, Quartz, Spangolite
  balance and align: Anandalite, Quartz
  spin too rapid/stuck open: Flint, Granite, Hematite
  spin too sluggish/stuck open: Quartz, Spangolite
  Note: any crystal will open the palm chakras.

Past life chakras: Ammolite, Astraline, Black Moonstone, Blizzard Stone, Brandenberg Amethyst, Catlinite, Chrysotile, Chrysotile in Serpentine, Coprolite, Cuprite with Chrysocolla, Dinosaur Bone, Dumortierite, Ethiopian Opal, Fire and Ice, Flint, Keyiapo, Larvikite, Lemurian Aquatine Calcite, Madagascar Quartz, Mystic Merlinite, Oceanite (Blue Onyx), Peanut Wood, Petrified Wood, Preseli Bluestone, Rainbow Mayanite, Rainbow Moonstone, Reinerite, Rhodozite, Rhyolite, Scheelite, Serpentine in Obsidian, Shiva Lingam, Smoky Amethyst, Tangerose, Tantalite, Titanite, Variscite, Violane (Blue Dioptase), Voegesite, Wind Fossil Agate
  balance and align: Dumortierite, Picasso Jasper, Rainbow Mayanite, Tangerose, Titanite, Violane (Blue Dioptase)
  spin too rapid/stuck open: Black Moonstone,

Coprolite, Flint, Petrified Wood, Preseli Bluestone, Sea Sediment Jasper, Scheelite, Tantalite

spin too sluggish/stuck closed: Blizzard Stone, Dragon Stone, Dumortierite, Garnet in Quartz, Rhodozite, Serpentine in Obsidian, Tantalite

Physical, subtle body: Amechlorite, Anandalite, Ancestralite, Bloodstone, Brandenberg Amethyst, Carnelian, Cradle of Life Stone, Dumortierite, Eilat Stone, Eklogite, Flint, Hematite, Kambaba Jasper, Madagascan Red 'Celestial Quartz', Quantum Quattro, Que Sera, Rainbow Mayanite, Red Amethyst, Sea Foam Flint, Stromatolite. *Chakra:* base, sacral, dantien, earth star

Planetary body: Aswan Granite, Brandenberg Amethyst, Charoite, Lapis Lazuli, Libyan Gold Tektite, Moldavite, Nebula Stone, Preseli Bluestone, Rainbow Mayanite, Starseed Quartz, Tektite. *Chakra:* past life, alta major, causal vortex, soma, stellar and Gaia gateway chakras

– S –

Sacral chakra: Amber, Amphibole, Bastnasite, Black Opal, Blue Jasper, Blue-green Fluorite, Blue-green Turquoise, Bumble Bee Jasper, Carnelian, Chinese Red Quartz, Citrine, Clinohumite, Golden and iron-coated Green Ridge Quartz, Golden Healer Quartz, Keyiapo, Limonite, Mahogany Obsidian, Orange Calcite, Orange Carnelian, Orange Kyanite, Orange Zincite, Realgar and Orpiment, Red Amethyst, Red Jasper, Red/Orange Zincite, Tangerose, Topaz, Triplite, Vanadinite

balance and align: Anandalite, Celestobarite, Golden

Healer Quartz, Green Ridge Quartz

spin too rapid/stuck open: Amber, Black Opal, Blue-green Fluorite, Blue-green Turquoise

spin too sluggish/stuck closed: Carnelian, Orange Zincite, Topaz, Triplite

Solar plexus chakra: Calcite, Citrine, Citrine Herkimer, Golden Azeztulite, Golden Beryl, Golden Calcite, Golden Coracalcite, Golden Danburite, Golden Enhydro, Golden Healer, Golden Labradorite (Bytownite), Green Chrysoprase, Green Prehnite, Green Ridge Quartz, Jasper, Libyan Glass Tektite, Light Green Hiddenite, Malachite, Obsidian, Rainbow Obsidian, Rhodochrosite, Rhodozite, Smoky Quartz, Sunstone, Tangerine Aura Quartz, Tangerine Dream Lemurian Seed, Tiger's Eye, Yellow Tourmaline, Yellow Zincite

balance and align: Anandalite, Citrine, Lemurian Seed

spin too rapid/stuck open: Calcite, Light Green Hiddenite, Malachite, Rainbow Obsidian, Smoky Quartz

spin too sluggish/stuck closed: Golden Calcite, Golden Danburite, Tangerine Aura Quartz, Yellow Labradorite (Bytownite)

Soma chakra: Afghanite, Amechlorite, Angelinite, Angel's Wing Calcite, Astraline, Auralite 23, Azeztulite, Banded Agate, Brandenberg Amethyst, Champagne Aura Quartz, Crystal Cap Amethyst, Diaspore (Zultanite), Faden Quartz, Fire and Ice, Holly Agate, Ilmenite, Isis Calcite, Lemurian Aquatine Calcite,

Merkabite Calcite, Natrolite, Nuummite, Owyhee Blue
Opal, Pentagonite, Petalite, Phantom Calcite, Phenacite
on Fluorite, Preseli Bluestone, Red Amethyst, Sacred
Scribe, Satyaloka and Satyamani Quartz, Scolecite,
Sedona Stone, Shaman Quartz, Stellar Beam Calcite,
Trigonic Quartz, Violane, Z-stone

> **balance and align:** Bytownite, Diaspore, Stellar Beam
> Calcite, Violane
>
> **spin too rapid/stuck open:** Isis Calcite, Pinky-beige
> Ussingite, Sedona Stone, Shaman Quartz, White
> Banded Agate
>
> **spin too sluggish/stuck closed:** Banded Agate,
> Diaspore, Nuummite, Preseli Bluestone

Soul Star chakra: Afghanite, Ajoite, Amethyst Elestial,
Amphibole, Anandalite, Angel's Wing Calcite,
Apophyllite, Astraline, Auralite 23, Azeztulite, Blue Flint,
Brandenberg Amethyst, Celestite, Celestobarite, Chevron
Amethyst, Citrine, Danburite, Dianite, Diaspore
(Zultanite), Elestial Quartz, Fire and Ice, Fire and Ice and
Nirvana Quartz, Golden Enhydro Herkimer, Golden
Himalayan Azeztulite, Green Ridge Quartz, Hematite,
Herkimer Diamond, Holly Agate, Keyiapo,
Khutnohorite, Kunzite, Lapis Lazuli, Lavender Quartz,
Merkabite Calcite, Muscovite, Natrolite, Novaculite,
Nuummite, Onyx, Orange River Quartz, Petalite,
Phenacite, Phenacite in Feldspar, Prophecy Stone, Purple
Siberian Quartz, Purpurite, Quartz, Rainbow Mayanite,
Rosophia, Satyamani and Satyaloka Quartz, Scolecite,
Selenite, Shungite, Snowflake Obsidian, Spirit Quartz,

Stellar Beam Calcite, Sugilite, Tangerine Aura Quartz, Tanzanite, Tanzine Aura Quartz, Titanite (Sphene), Trigonic Quartz, Vera Cruz Amethyst, Violane, White Elestial

> **balance and align:** Anandalite, Vera Cruz Amethyst, Violane
>
> **spin too rapid/stuck open:** Celestobarite, Novaculite, Nuummite, Pinky-beige Ussingite, White, Rose or Smoky Elestial Quartz
>
> **spin too sluggish/stuck closed:** Golden Himalayan Azeztulite, Petalite, Phenacite, Rosophia

Spiritual body: Anandalite, Azeztulite, Brandenberg Amethyst, Golden Herkimer Diamond, Golden Quartz, Green Ridge Quartz, Larimar, Lemurian Seed, Nirvana Quartz, Phenacite, Rainbow Mayanite, Shaman Quartz, Trigonic Amethyst, Trigonic Quartz. *Chakra:* past life, soul star, stellar gateway, alta major, causal vortex

Spleen chakra: Amber, Aventurine, Bloodstone, Carnelian, Charoite, Chlorite Quartz, Emerald, Eye of the Storm, Fire Opal, Flint, Gaspeite, Green Fluorite, Jade, Orange River Quartz, Prasiolite, Rhodochrosite, Rhodonite, Ruby, Tugtupite, Zircon

> **balance and align:** Charoite, Emerald, Eye of the Storm, Flint, Green Aventurine, Tugtupite
>
> **clear attachments and hooks:** Aventurine, Chert, Flint, Gaspeite, Jade, Jasper, Lemurian Seed
>
> **for the right armpit:** Bloodstone, Eye of the Storm, Gaspeite, Triplite, Tugtupite
>
> **spin too rapid/stuck open:** Amber, Aventurine,

Chlorite Quartz, Eye of the Storm, Flint, Gaspeite, Green Fluorite, Jade, Prasiolite, Tugtupite

spin too sluggish/stuck closed: Fire Opal, Orange River Quartz, Rhodonite, Ruby, Topaz

Stellar gateway chakra: Afghanite, Ajoite, Amethyst Elestial, Amphibole, Anandalite™, Angelinite, Angel's Wing Calcite, Apophyllite, Astraline, Azeztulite, Brandenberg Amethyst, Celestite, Dianite, Diaspore (Zultanite), Elestial Quartz, Fire and Ice, Golden Himalayan Azeztulite, Golden Selenite, Green Ridge Quartz, Holly Agate, Ice Quartz, Kunzite, Merkabite Calcite, Moldavite, Nirvana Quartz, Novaculite, Petalite, Phenacite, Purpurite, Stellar Beam Calcite, Titanite (Sphene), Trigonic Quartz, White Elestial Quartz

balance and align: Ajoite, Amethyst Elestial, Anandalite, Brandenberg Amethyst, Kunzite

spin too rapid/stuck open: Amphibole Quartz, Ice Quartz, Merkabite Calcite, Pinky-beige Ussingite, Purpurite

spin too sluggish/stuck closed: Angel's Wing Calcite, Disaspore, Phenacite

– T –

Third eye (brow) chakra: Afghanite, Ajo Quartz, Ajoite, Amber, Amechlorite, Amethyst, Ammolite, Amphibole Quartz, Angelite, Apophyllite, Aquamarine, Axinite, Azurite, Black Moonstone, Blue Calcite, Blue Kyanite, Blue Lace Agate, Blue Obsidian, Blue Selenite, Blue Topaz, Blue Tourmaline, Bytownite (Yellow Labradorite),

Cacoxenite, Cavansite, Champagne Aura Quartz, Diaspore, Electric-blue Obsidian, Eye of the Storm, Garnet, Glaucophane, Golden Himalayan Azeztulite, Herderite, Herkimer Diamond, Holly Agate, Howlite, Indigo Auram, Iolite, Kunzite, Labradorite, Lapis Lazuli, Lavender-purple Opal, Lazulite, Lepidolite, Libyan Gold Tektite, Malachite with Azurite (use as polished stone, create essence by indirect method), Moldavite, Pietersite, Purple Fluorite, Rhomboid Selenite, Sapphire, Serpentine in Obsidian, Sodalite, Spectrolite, Stilbite, Sugilite, Tangerine Aura Quartz, Turquoise, Unakite, Yellow Labradorite (Bytownite)

> **balance and align:** Anandalite, Sugilite
>
> **spin too rapid/stuck open:** Diaspore, Iolite, Lavender-purple Opal, Pietersite, Serpentine in Obsidian, Sodalite, Sugilite
>
> **spin too sluggish/stuck closed:** Apophyllite, Azurite, Banded Agate, Diaspore, Herkimer Diamond, Optical Calcite, Rhomboid Calcite, Rhomboid Selenite, Royal Blue Sapphire, Tanzine Aura Quartz, Yellow Labradorite (Bytownite)

Throat chakra: Ajo Quartz, Ajoite, Amber, Amethyst, Aquamarine, Astraline, Azurite, Blue Chalcedony, Blue Kyanite, Blue Lace Agate, Blue Obsidian, Blue Quartz, Blue Topaz, Blue Tourmaline, Chalcanthite, Chrysocolla, Chrysotile, Eye of the Storm, Glaucophane, Green Ridge Quartz, Indicolite Quartz, Kunzite, Lapis Lace, Lapis Lazuli, Lepidolite, Moldavite, Paraiba Tourmaline, Sugilite, Turquoise

balance and align: Anandalite, Blue Chalcedony, Blue Lace Agate, Blue Topaz, Indicolite Quartz, Sapphire
spin too rapid/stuck open: Black Sapphire, Lepidolite, Paraiba Tourmaline, Sugilite, Turquoise
spin too sluggish/stuck closed: Chrysocolla, Lapis Lazuli, Moldavite, Turquoise

"Always use ethically sourced Coral.

Part V: Astrological and Astral-Magic Essences

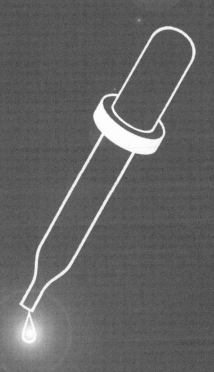

A highly versatile tool, astrology can help you to know yourself fully. From an astrologer's point of view, the map of the heavens at the moment of birth, known as the natal or birthchart, is a map of the psyche. But astrology is much more than this... The art of astrology lies in bringing together the different components of the birthchart into a coherent whole.

– Astrology Bible, Judy Hall

A natal or birthchart is a moment fixed in time. A picture of the sky as it appears from the perspective of earth *at that time and place* against the ecliptic – the sun's path around the heavens. That path is divided into twelve segments: the signs of the zodiac. And, yes, Western astrologers do recognise that the precession of the equinoxes has occurred (changing the current astronomical background), but we prefer to use a fixed background that harks back to the origins of astrology. The planets and signs in the birthchart map out the soul's learning plan for the present lifetime. Challenges and issues can be assisted to resolve, and the gifts brought out, by creating an astrological essence.

Many of the crystals and gems associated with the zodiac and with the hours of the day and night, days of the week and months of the year have their basis in ancient astral-magic. As sources vary in their attributions, a choice of crystals is almost always available. Dowse for those most suitable for your purpose when creating the essence.

The Zodiac

The sun travels along the ecliptic (sun's path) across the heavens at roughly the same time each year, although it may vary by a day or so. This gives rise to the zodiac signs. The planets move across that background, giving rise to an individual birthchart.

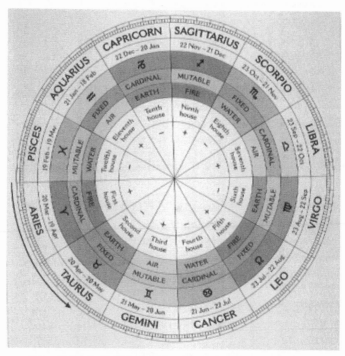

The Zodiac Wheel, signs, elements and qualities

Correspondence

According to ancient traditions spanning several thousand years, certain crystals are associated with specific zodiac signs or planets. But, as with birthstones, there is no 'one-size-fits-all'. Many crystals are involved. The correspondences differ because the links between signs and planets and crystals were determined in the distant past by various sources: Mesopotamian, Egyptian, Greek, Vedic, Chinese, Arabic and so on. The traditions migrated as people travelled the ancient world. Birthstones, for instance, may arise from Western or Eastern cosmology, and from esoteric or exoteric traditions. These are often, but not necessarily, linked to the 'planetary ruler' of the sign. This book incorporates these alternatives into the companion crystals for a sign. The birthstones themselves have been chosen on the basis of astrological association, compatibility, and the life-enhancing qualities the crystals offer. For some signs, two birthstones are listed. In these cases, the two crystals balance and harmonise each other, each offering a much needed quality to the sign (*see The Crystal Zodiac for further details*).

As the signs are associated with different spheres of life, you can use essences for a sign to assist you with specific issues. If, for instance, you have partnership problems, you can turn to Libra, the relationship sign. Here you will discover crystals for all facets of relationship. Libra is a diplomatic sign and you will also find appropriate crystals for resolving conflict and for facilitating decision making.

The soul's journey around the zodiac is an ancient concept. The soul experiences different facets of life in each sign:

Aries: "I am". Personality, ego, Self, physical appearance, action, assertiveness, how others perceive you.

Taurus: "I possess". Values, personal possessions, self-worth, inner security, the material world.

Gemini: "I communicate". Mental activity, knowledge, intuition, short journeys, siblings, early education.

Cancer: "I feel". Nurturing, emotions, roots, mother, home and family, tradition, possessiveness.

Leo: "I shine": Creative expression, recognition, heart-centredness, personal power, children.

Virgo: "I analyse". Service, physical health, intellectualism, diet, co-workers, analysis, attention to detail, perfection.

Libra: "We are". Relationships, commitment, balance, fairness, judgement, fair play, harmony.

Scorpio: "I desire". Death, rebirth and transformation, mysteries, secrets, sex, mysticism, taboo areas.

Sagittarius: "I teach". Questions and questing, higher education, philosophy, religion, law, the bigger picture, long-distance travel, optimism, expansion.

Capricorn: "I consolidate". Career, material reality, social persona, authority figures, crone-wisdom, judgement, scapegoat.

Aquarius: "I think". Humanitarianism, foresight,

ideals, hopes, friendship, rebellion, eccentricity.

Pisces: "I merge". Mysticism, illumination, enlight-
enment, compassion, collective unconscious, fantasy,
karma, self-deception, psychic sensitivity, escapism.

Reading the chart glyphs

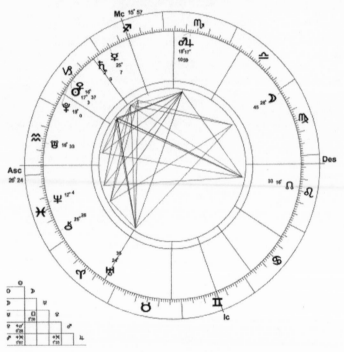

The zodiac chart for the inception of this section.
Simply match the glyphs (symbols) for the signs and
planets – *and see page 134.*

The Zodiac Glyphs

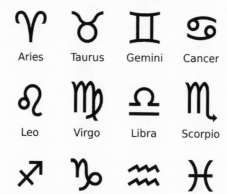

Aries	Taurus	Gemini	Cancer
Leo	Virgo	Libra	Scorpio
Sagittarius	Capricorn	Aquarius	Pisces

Planetary glyphs

⊙ Sun

☽ Moon

☿ Mercury

♀ Venus

♂ Mars

♃ Jupiter

⚷ Chiron

♄ Saturn

♅ Uranus

♆ Neptune

♇ Pluto

☊ Node

Birthstones

Each sign traditionally has a birthstone attributed to it and a ruling planet that oversees the sign (*and see the Directory page 161*).

Sun Sign	Glyph	Birthstone(s)	Ruling Planet
Aries	♈	Ruby, Diamond	Mars
Taurus	♉	Emerald	Venus
Gemini	♊	Agate, Tourmaline	Mercury
Cancer	♋	Moonstone	Moon
Leo	♌	Cat's or Tiger's Eye	Sun
Virgo	♍	Peridot, Sardonyx	Mercury
Libra	♎	Sapphire, Opal	Venus
Scorpio	♏	Malachite, Turquoise	Pluto, Mars
Sagittarius	♐	Topaz, Turquoise	Jupiter
Capricorn	♑	Onyx, Garnet	Saturn
Aquarius	♒	Aquamarine	Uranus, Saturn
Pisces	♓	Amethyst	Neptune, Jupiter

The body and the Zodiac

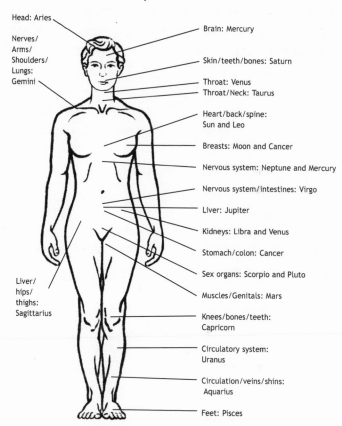

Head: Aries

Nerves/
Arms/
Shoulders/
Lungs:
Gemini

Brain: Mercury

Skin/teeth/bones: Saturn

Throat: Venus
Throat/Neck: Taurus

Heart/back/spine:
Sun and Leo

Breasts: Moon and Cancer

Nervous system: Neptune and Mercury

Nervous system/intestines: Virgo

Liver: Jupiter

Kidneys: Libra and Venus

Stomach/colon: Cancer

Sex organs: Scorpio and Pluto

Muscles/Genitals: Mars

Liver/
hips/
thighs:
Sagittarius

Knees/bones/teeth:
Capricorn

Circulatory system:
Uranus

Circulation/veins/shins:
Aquarius

Feet: Pisces

The body and zodiac sign correspondences (taken from
The Astrology Bible)

Using a crystal birthchart essence

Placing appropriate crystals on a chart harmonises it. But
rather than placing them on the chart, if you create an

essence from appropriate crystals you create a synergetic energy that balances all the parts. Either take or rub on the essence frequently, spray it around yourself, add it to your bathwater, or place a central crystal on the chart and drip the essence on to it. Create an essence to:

- Sedate an excess of an element in the chart (see below), use sedating stones for appropriate elemental signs.
- Strengthen a weak element by using strengthening crystals for the element that is lacking.
- Strengthen a challenged planet with appropriate crystals (see page 134).
- Harmonise a specific planetary pattern with appropriate crystals.
- Equalize the planetary effects with an appropriate crystal for each.
- Regard the signs as 'chakras' (see page 135) and use appropriately coloured crystals for 'missing' signs (i.e. signs that do not have planets located in them) when creating the essence.
- As there is a correlation between the zodiac and parts of the body, appropriate crystals can be added to physiological essences and rubbed over the site where appropriate.

Balancing the elements

Zodiac signs belong to one of four 'elements'. The elements filter and regulate the energy of the planets. The number of planets in an element is generally shown in a box below the chart, or, if the chart is coloured, will be indicated by colour. If your chart doesn't indicate how many planets are in each element, you can count them for yourself using the zodiac wheel on page 132. Each element is related to a particular function of the overall self: Earth to the body and matter, Water to the emotions and emotional intuition, Air to the mind, and Fire to the spirit and intuition. The balance of planets within each element describes how much at ease within these specific realms of experience a person is. Some charts will be well balanced with an equal number of planets in each element. Others may be imbalanced with one or no planets in a particular element and a large number in another.

The elements each represent a different way of perceiving life. Earth is practical and sense-orientated. It perceives the world through eyes, ears, nose, mouth and touch. Water has a sensitivity and feeling perception that experiences the world through subtle sensing and emotion. The Air element is the intellectual element, understanding through thought and logical reason, whilst the Fire element is intuitive and knowing. The number of planets placed in each element shapes behaviour, indicating how the person perceives reality. Strong emphasis on one or two elements leads to a deficiency in others and specific combinations of elements give rise to a characteristic approach to the world.

Whilst a balanced number of planets in all the elements tends to favour expression of the element in which the Sun is placed, a preponderance of an element that is not harmonious with the sun-sign can powerfully affect how the Sun is expressed, particularly if the Moon or Mars is placed in the prominent element. Fortunately the elemental balance can be redressed by a calming crystal essence for the predominant element(s), and a strengthening essence for the deficient element(s).

Fire-Earth

When working well, this combination has enormous staying power as the fiery energy is harnessed and earthed towards practical tasks. If the combination is not working well and Earth overly restricts Fire, then a sudden explosion results.

Fire-Air

A volatile combination prone to explosive bursts of energy followed by burnout or mental exhaustion. This combination is happy in the realm of ideas and imagination but finds it difficult to live in the everyday world.

Fire-Water

When Fire and Water come together, the emotions tend to overheat. The lively energy of Fire can be quenched by excess emotion but the combination can be intuitive and imaginative.

Earth-Air

Air and Earth tend not to mix well together, as the slow and orderly processes of Earth are anathema to Air. However, this combination can lead to sustained and productive thought.

Air-Water

With this combination, people tend to live in the imagination, or to have their head in the clouds. There are many ideas, mostly impractical, but this is a poetic combination as it puts feelings into words.

Earth-Water

This combination can be dull and solid, or productive and hard working. Earth tends to muddy Water, restricting emotional expression and creating misunderstandings.

Element imbalances

The overall balance of the elements within a chart can indicate subtle dis-ease, depletion or excess, that can be brought into equilibrium with crystal essences. Imbalances may be innate – the birthchart – or temporary, such as progressed charts or solar returns and strong transits (the current movements of the planets activating a specific point in the birthchart). If you know something about astrology you could create a transit or progression essence. Transits may be long or short duration. If you don't know anything about astrology, you'll often get a clue from reading your horoscope and seeing remarks such as "with Saturn entering your sign for a two-year stay..." or, much shorter term, Mercury, Venus or Mars. The imbalance can equally apply to a large number or a small number of planets in an element highlighting issues.

The Elements

Earth: *Issue:* abused or ignored body or too body- and materialism-orientated, toxicity. *Depleted Earth:* weakness, incohesion, fractures/blockages/breaks on any level that fail to heal, abuse. Poverty or a sense of lack in the family line. *Excess Earth:* resists change, obesity, blockages, depression, ossification, calcification, and loss of acuity of senses. Over-materialism, holding on.

Water: *Issue:* emotion-logged or emotionally constipated. *Depleted Water:* results in thirst, dehydration, cramps, insomnia, poor memory, and inability to show feelings – sense of being drowned by family. *Excess Water:* creates mucus, pneumonia, fluid retention, obesity, clogged arteries, and lymphatic retention. Over-emotionality, family secrets.

Air: *Issue:* mental emphasis (excess) or senses emphasis (lack). *Weakened Air:* poor communication or circulation, lack of self-confidence, despondency, nightmares, nausea, toxicity, oxygen deficiency, shortness of breath and fatigue – feeling of being smothered. *Excess Air:* creates nervous disorders, restlessness, hypersensitivity to pollutants, harsh sounds and odours; autism, rough skin, brittle hair, bones and nails, flatulence, asthma, coughs, constipation, insomnia, schizophrenia, arthritis and rough skin. Difficulty fitting into environment.

Fire: *Issue:* intuition, over-impulsive, energetic burnout. *Depleted Fire:* low vitality, despondency, loss of appetite, pallor, cold, slow and inadequate digestion, migraine, phobias, low immunity, poor circulation and muscle tone, possible diabetes. Overbearing/bullying parenting. *Excess Fire:* uncontrolled anger and aggression, heartburn, liver and gallbladder problems, digestive complaints, ulcers, excess bile, fever, skin eruptions, a tendency to body odour, blurred vision and hypoglycaemia. Abuse, anger/aggression passing down the ancestral line.

For crystals, see Elemental imbalances page 171.

The luminaries and the planets

The Sun

In astrological terms the Sun is your Self, what you are building into the present. In some systems of astrology it is your character but the deeper meaning behind it is the soul qualities that your soul intends to develop. It is also the father. Choose two or three crystals from the list below that applies to your Sun. Each sun-sign approaches the world in a specific way that an essence will either strengthen or mitigate.

The Moon

In astrological terms, the Moon is your intuition, your past, your emotions, your comfort zone – and your mother. Your intuition can be strengthened by an appropriate crystal essence for the Moon placement in your birthchart, and underlying Moon issues rectified.

The North and South Nodes

As the North and South Nodes are always opposite each other, with the North Node indicating your present soul purpose and your South Node your past soul purpose and soul gifts already gained, you can use the solar crystals for the sign in which your North Node is positioned and lunar crystals for the South Node in addition to the crystals in the A-Z directory.

Planetary strengths

Sun: vitality, courage, self-worth.

Moon: compassion, caring, intuition.

Mercury: perceptive insight, good communication.

Venus: ability to love, appropriate values, aesthetics.

Mars: willpower and assertiveness, 'can-do' attitude.

Jupiter: expansion, faith, optimism.

Saturn: consolidation, karmic knowledge, crone-wisdom, good boundaries, grounded.

Chiron: healing abilities.

Uranus: foresight, catalyst, transformation.

Neptune: metaphysical insight, intuitive, caring.

Pluto: survival, capacity to go where others fear to tread, transformation.

Planetary weaknesses

Sun: attitudes such as former arrogance/pride, tendency passes through father. *Fire-sun:* burns out easily. *Earth-sun:* energy goes into work. *Water-sun:* emotional overload. *Air-sun:* too head-orientated.

Moon: heredity and reproduction problems, ingrained toxic emotions.

Mercury: ingrained mental issues and beliefs create disease, scattered thought processes, pernickityness.

Venus: toxic relationship patterns, values are skewed.

Mars: old rage, aggression, too timid, old injuries, attitudes.

Jupiter: overindulgence, body image (earth signs).

Saturn: rigidity, fear, judgementalism, authoritarianism.

Chiron: wounds to the physical body, psyche and soul.

Uranus: vibrational misalignment.

Neptune: picks up 'outside influences', psychic sponge, old allergies, non-alignment of physical and etheric results in endocrine disturbance.

Pluto: deep-seated, abuse, anger, sexual problems.

For crystals see the Directory.

Challenging aspects

Aspects are the relationships planets make with one another across and around a chart – signified by the lines in the centre of the example chart. Some aspects are harmonious, others can be challenging as they unify or bring the planetary energies into conflict. Some depend on how you use them, which is where crystal essences come in. This is a layer of the chart that could perhaps be left to those who can read a birthchart, but if you intuit

that a strong line connecting two planets, or two or more planets placed side by side or at right angles to each other, could be challenging or beneficial, by all means find an appropriate crystal for those planets and create an essence. Drip it into the centre of the chart or, better still, place a clear Quartz or Flint in the centre and drip the essence on to that.

Astral-magic

Astral-magic is particularly useful for timing the creation of essences. Talismans were traditionally created and spells carried out according to the planetary hour, the day of the week or month of the year. These ancient crystal connections can be harnessed to your essence-making, particularly for abundance and aspirational essences (see page 180).

Planetary days and hours

It is possible to create astrological essences utilising the ancient system of 'planetary days and hours'. The hours start at sunrise, rather than in the modern system of midnight, and go around to sunrise the following day. 'Day' begins at sunrise and ends at sunset. 'Night' begins at sunset and ends at sunrise. Not surprising as the system began with Chaldean astrologers who enjoyed virtually equal and constant-in-length days and nights. The further north or south you travel from the equator the more the days and nights lengthen and shorten, of course. And, to further complicate matters, the hours are not of equal length. This can make essence creation according to the planetary hours a trifle complex to say the least, although online tables are available that also take account of your location (see Resources). However, the system of the seven traditional 'planets' ruling days of the week is an easy one to follow (while not planets in the astronomical sense, the luminaries, the sun and moon, are referred to as planets in astrology). Simply begin creating your essence at or after sunrise on the day of the week ruled by the planet to capture its influence. If you are working with the less traditional, more recently discovered planets, you can use the 'higher octave' principle to pair these with the traditional planets.

The planetary days

Sunday: Sun
Monday: Moon
Tuesday: Mars, Pluto
Wednesday: Mercury, Uranus
Thursday: Jupiter, Chiron
Friday: Venus, Neptune
Saturday: Saturn

See page 173 for crystals for the days of the week and page 176 for months of the year.

Planetary Hours of the Day

Hour	Sunday	Monday	Tuesday	Wednesday	Thursday	Friday	Saturday
1	Sun	Moon	Mars	Mercury	Jupiter	Venus	Saturn
2	Venus	Saturn	Sun	Moon	Mars	Mercury	Jupiter
3	Mercury	Jupiter	Venus	Saturn	Sun	Moon	Mars
4	Moon	Mars	Mercury	Jupiter	Venus	Saturn	Sun
5	Saturn	Sun	Moon	Mars	Mercury	Jupiter	Venus
6	Jupiter	Venus	Saturn	Sun	Moon	Mars	Mercury
7	Mars	Mercury	Jupiter	Venus	Saturn	Sun	Moon
8	Sun	Moon	Mars	Mercury	Jupiter	Venus	Saturn
9	Venus	Saturn	Sun	Moon	Mars	Mercury	Jupiter
10	Mercury	Jupiter	Venus	Saturn	Sun	Moon	Mars
11	Moon	Mars	Mercury	Jupiter	Venus	Saturn	Sun
12	Saturn	Sun	Moon	Mars	Mercury	Jupiter	Venus

Planetary Hours of the Night

Hours	Sunday	Monday	Tuesday	Wednesday	Thursday	Friday	Saturday
1	Jupiter	Venus	Saturn	Sun	Moon	Mars	Mercury
2	Mars	Mercury	Jupiter	Venus	Saturn	Sun	Moon
3	Sun	Moon	Mars	Mercury	Jupiter	Venus	Saturn
4	Venus	Saturn	Sun	Moon	Mars	Mercury	Jupiter
5	Mercury	Jupiter	Venus	Saturn	Sun	Moon	Mars
6	Moon	Mars	Mercury	Jupiter	Venus	Saturn	Sun
7	Saturn	Sun	Moon	Mars	Mercury	Jupiter	Venus
8	Jupiter	Venus	Saturn	Sun	Moon	Mars	Mercury
9	Mars	Mercury	Jupiter	Venus	Saturn	Sun	Moon
10	Sun	Moon	Mars	Mercury	Jupiter	Venus	Saturn
11	Venus	Saturn	Sun	Moon	Mars	Mercury	Jupiter
12	Mercury	Jupiter	Venus	Saturn	Sun	Moon	Mars

Taken from Henry Cornelius Agrippa's *Three Books of Occult Philosophy*

Note: See the Directory for crystals for the hours of the day and night, days of the week and months of the year.

The fixed stars and star systems

The upper heaven is Luladanitu stone of Anu [supreme sky god]. He settled the 300 Igigu [gods of heaven] inside.

The middle heaven is Saggilmut stone of the Igigu. Bel [Jupiter] sat on a throne within on a dais of lapis lazuli. He made glass and crystal shine inside.

The lower heaven is jasper of the stars. He drew constellations of the gods on it.

– Assyrian text, Alasdair Livingstone[5]

At one time the ancients believed that the sky was

actually a set of nested crystal spheres on to which were hung the luminaries, planets and stars. While modern science has shown this to be a fallacy, the connection between stars, crystals and the firmament has remained. The sun moves along the ecliptic against a background of fixed stars, celestial bodies such as dwarf planets and asteroids, and the constellations. A constellation is a group of stars forming a recognisable pattern. The signs of the zodiac are constellations but there are other stellar constellations that have been recognised since ancient times.

A fixed star appears as part of a constellation and remains constant, as a luminous point, relative to other celestial bodies, in contrast to the planets, the 'wandering stars' that change position at speeds that differ according to their orbit around the sun and, at times, even appearing to go backwards in the sky. Some astrologers, ancient and modern, utilise the fixed stars in their inter-pretation of the sky or for timing rituals. In other words, for divination and magic. The energy of the fixed stars, celestial bodies and constellations can be harnessed using crystals. This is essence making for those with specialised knowledge and interest, but it can be used, if you wish, to contact beings from certain star systems such as the Pleiades, or individual stars such as Sirius, for instance, or to feel in touch with your 'home star'. (See Resources for fixed star lists available online, and the directory for crystals allied to star systems.)

Would you like an example?

At this stage, an example or two will no doubt assist in understanding the zodiac and planets at a deeper level and offer insight into the process of applying the crystals for assistance.

Example 1: **Counteracting Saturnine conditions**

So, for an example of how a planetary crystal essence could work, let's look for a moment at counteracting typical issues that arise either from a weak or dominant natal Saturn, or during a transit – the passage of a planet in the current sky through a sign making a contact with planets in your own birthchart. At the time of writing, Saturn has recently changed signs from Sagittarius to Capricorn, its own sign. So the influence is particularly powerful and will radiate through all the earth element signs. Saturn can be a challenge indicating potential blockages, rigidity and stonewalls – especially around following the accepted mores of a society. But it's also karmic and ancestral wisdom to be accessed and put into practice in the modern world (see the example chart page 151) and it is the planet of steady progress and consolidation with a flair for long-term forward planning. An essence made from a selection of the following crystals could input counterbalancing energies to dissolve blockages and reveal the wisdom:

Agate or Onyx: the strength and persistence to work

through blockages.

Agrellite: heals the inner saboteur.

Anandalite: brings celestial light and divine guidance into the situation.

Aquamarine: overcomes judgementalism and authoritarianism.

Blue Scapolite: heals self-sabotage.

Epidote: heals the inner critic.

Galena: (*caution: toxic*) brings balance on all levels, dissolving self-limiting beliefs from the past.

Hematite: grounds, harmonises, assists with maintaining sensible boundaries.

Magnetite: overcomes extreme rigidity or stiffness.

Selenite: brings lightness and the higher divine, more spiritual side of Saturn to the fore.

Example 2: **Creating a birthchart essence**

A birthchart can be created for any moment in time, not just a physical birth. It works for projects too. So, this chart is for the inception of the astrological section in this book. The moment when I sat down to actually write it, gathering together the information and getting it down on the computer, instead of having vague ideas floating around my head. Naturally, as soon as I printed the chart, I placed crystals on it. It was a Sunday, harnessing the brightest possibilities of the sun.

These crystals would be made into an essence for the book when the sun shone again – I was writing during a particularly grey period of winter. Which was totally appropriate given how much Capricorn energy was present in the chart. Excellent for long-term planning and creating solid foundations. But not for immediate implementation. However, ten days later, the sun was

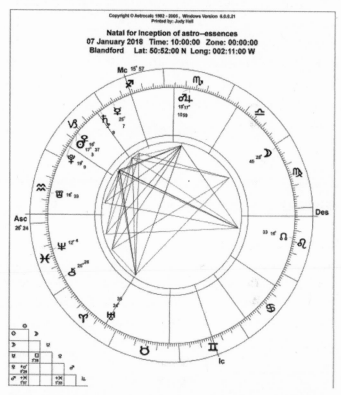

shining brightly so the essence was set out on a lump of Celtic Quartz in the sun and, as it was a new moon, the essence would incorporate those energies too together with the heightened intuitive and transmutative commu-nication of Mercury and Uranus as it was bottled on a

Wednesday: their day. As you'll see in a moment, all the elements made themselves felt as the essence was being created. A piece of grandmother wisdom came my way too, courtesy of Terrie Celest of www.astrology wise.co.uk.

> *The grandmothers, their connection with and concern for Mother Earth, their new way of walking on it, their feminine energies, give Saturn the lightness that was missing. Anything that has an Earth connection, has to have a strong feminine connection too.*
> – Capricorn new moon newsletter

It perfectly underlined what the essence was doing: resolving the contradictions of a feminine, 'negative', earth sign, Capricorn, being ruled by the coldest sternest planet, Saturn, and answering the question of how do you get to, and utilise, the wisdom at the heart of the sign (see below). Perfect! The essence will be dropped on to the keystone in the centre until the book is published.

Salient points of the chart

The planets and signs

Extremely strong emphasis on Capricorn energy:

  Saturn in Capricorn
  Sun in Capricorn   ) three planets in conjunction,
  Venus in Capricorn) that is next to each other
  Pluto in Capricorn   )

Moon in Virgo: throwing light on underlying psychosomatics.

Mercury in Sagittarius: bringing much needed clarity to the process.

Mars and Jupiter conjunct in Scorpio: digging deep for transformation.

Chiron and Neptune in Pisces: possibly clouding the issue of deep wounds to the spiritual self but also indicating a desire to escape back from incarnation into oneness. The positive side of this would be to expand consciousness.

Uranus in Aries: total transformation of the Self and revolutionary new methods.

North Node in Leo, South Node in Aquarius: the need to shine out the true Self and own your own power.

Elemental imbalance

There is an imbalance of elements in the chart. No planets in air. Five planets in earth. Two in fire. If we count the wounded-healer planet Chiron (which is not shown on element lists), there are four planets in water. The planets in earth are grounding the writing, but the lack of air planets along with the foggy planet Neptune being the first planet you meet on the journey around the chart (a chart is read anticlockwise) means that finding clarity is challenging. There is plenty of intuition at work but structure could be lacking. The shape of the chart is an upside-down 'bowl', reflecting our thoughts inward to discover the core truth of the chart.

The aspects

Perhaps the biggest challenge and the key to unlocking the whole lies in harmonising the energy of the two 'angels wings' triangles that radiate from the Mars-Jupiter conjunction. One 'wing' the triangle of Uranus opposite Jupiter-Mars and Sun-Pluto-Venus and the other 'wing' the triangle of Venus-Sun-Pluto inconjunct the North Node also radiating from Mars-Jupiter. It has enormous potential for transformation, whatever Jupiter can envisage it can bring into being, but also for challenging entrenched authority figures and fixed saturnine mores. The lore and legislation around essences is a minefield that has to be trodden with care. And, the 'photographic method' could be unacceptable to some traditional essence practitioners, although precedents are being set with flower essence photographs as new vibrational understanding develops.

The challenge

Translating astrological concepts into words that a reader new to astrology could understand requires the mind to be functioning in a particular way. Fortunately all that Capricorn energy is extremely structure-orientated, but that structure is tradition-led. We are breaking through old boundaries here to transform energies and introduce new concepts. The crystals for reaching elemental balance and many of those for the planets arise out of my findings over fifty years of working with crystals, essences and charts rather than from 'traditional' astrology or essence creation.

And a different face of Capricorn could be brought out through utilising the potential of Saturn in its own sign:

Any planet that is in its own sign, has the opportunity to work at its best, to express its full potential and for us to tap into its positive expression as well as the negative one. It doesn't mean that we won't have challenges from it, but that the positive, higher expression of that planet can be accessed more easily than at any other time; we can find the gift, turn it around and find a positive expression.

– Terrie Celest, www.astrologywise.co.uk, January new moon newsletter

The crystal remedy

First of all, that element imbalance was addressed. Placing an Aquamarine on Mercury in Sagittarius helped me to define the underlying organising principles behind the zodiac and it also harnessed the emotional intuition signified by all the water planets to the active intuition of the fire element. It also activated the transformatory energies of catalytic Uranus. Mercury in Sagittarius always asks the fundamental question, 'What does it mean?' Aquamarine and Uranus give the answer: look to the spiritual dimension – and the unexpected. Filtering information reaching the brain and clarifying perception, Aquamarine dissolves self-defeating programmes allowing the soul's voice to be heard. Selenite on the Moon in Virgo assisted with not only bringing more 'divine light' into the situation but also triggered the soul-gift of having already learned how to analyse and discern. The Capricorn energies were harnessed using Ancestralite. Bringing in the wisdom of the ancestors, harnessing tradition to transmutation (Pluto).

Synchronistically, the new-moon-in-Capricorn newsletter from Terrie Celest of www.astrologywise arrived in my in-box just as the sun shone brightly and I could finally create the essence. The newsletter was all about Saturn in Capricorn and it may assist with understanding the energies involved and the point of change we had reached:

> Ironically, I [Terrie] wondered, with Saturn's association with tradition, are we actually viewing Saturn too traditionally? It felt almost as if he needs a software update for 2018! I questioned my own thoughts and feelings on

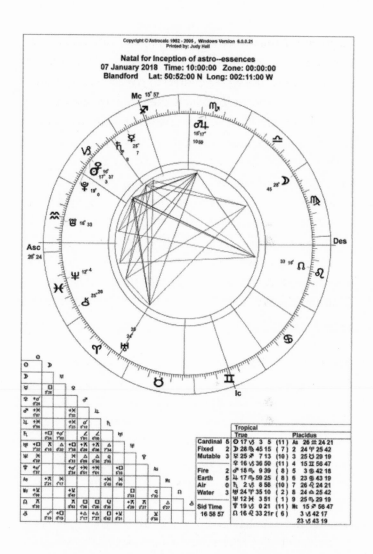

tradition and acknowledged that perhaps the rebel in me
[Uranus is strong in Terrie's chart] was squirming at the
word. I tried to think of the positive use of traditions… My

answer came through Gemini Brett, who was talking in [a] webinar about Saturn and Capricorn. His teacher of shamanic astrology, Daniel Giamario said Capricorn wasn't "about governments or beliefs, rule makers, law-giver, but is the council of grandmothers, of wise elders, Earth teachers who are here to preserve the traditions for 7 future generations." ...

Capricorn energies help us to connect to Earth wisdoms and traditions. That was my Ah-ha moment, something inside me resonated very deeply with those words, or rather, those words resonated and kindled, something deep inside. Council of grandmothers, Earth teachers, wisdom from the Earth not just from the ancestors, those words made me stop and think. A knowing, a re-kindling of old knowledge, a missing link that brought other pieces of my jigsaw of understanding together and gave me a new perspective... These wonderful grandmothers are blending tradition, the wisdom of tradition and the Earth into today, bringing a new way to walk it.

The International Council of Thirteen Indigenous Grandmothers, such a great expression of the feminine side of Capricorn. This from their website:

We, the International Council of Thirteen Indigenous Grandmothers, believe that our ancestral ways of prayer, peacemaking and healing are vitally needed today. We come together to nurture, educate and train our children. We come together to uphold the practice of our ceremonies and affirm the right to use our plant medicines free of legal restriction. We come together to protect our lands where our peoples live and upon which our cultures depend, to safeguard the collective heritage of traditional medicines, and to defend the earth Herself. We believe that the teachings of our ancestors will light our way through an uncertain future.

– www.grandmotherscouncil.org

An Ancestralite crystal grounded the energies in a way that allows transformation to take place without the negative side of Saturn in Capricorn digging its heels in to thwart change to an entrenched system. To activate the purpose and balance out the energies of the triangle, raw Iolite-and-Sunstone was added. A central keystone of Brandenberg Amethyst, a crystal with the purest, most refined of vibrations, supported the whole.

Elemental intervention: Creating the essence

The crystals stayed on the chart until a change in the weather meant an essence could be prepared. But putting the essence out in the sun was swiftly followed by a violent gust of wind and a short sharp shower, resulting in a rainbow. All within half an hour. So that was all the elements covered as the essence was standing on a huge piece of rock. The essence also captured the energies of the day's new moon. A final plutonian piece clicked in when Cleansing Service's poo-lorry (as my young granddaughters named it) arrived to empty the septic tank over the road. Perfect symbolism!

The essence for the chart: Ancestralite, Aquamarine, Iolite-and-Sunstone, Selenite. *Dropped on to the Brandenberg Amethyst, which remained on the centre of the chart.*

Directory: Crystals for astrological essences

Choose 1–4 crystals from an entry when creating your essence. Add a regulating crystal if appropriate.

– Solar crystals –

Solar crystals: Celtic Golden Quartz, Citrine, Golden Beryl, Golden Green Ridge or Arkansas Quartz, Golden Quartz, Golden Topaz, Goldstone, Rainbow Lattice Sunstone, Rainbow Mayanite, Ruby, Sulphur, Sunstone, Sunstone-and-Iolite, Zircon

> **Sun in Aries:** *Birthstones:* Diamond, Ruby. *Abundance Crystal:* Carnelian. *Ritual Crystal:* Fire Agate. *Companion Crystals:* Amethyst, Aquamarine, Aventurine, Bloodstone, Carnelian, Citrine, Fire Agate, Garnet, Iolite with Sunstone, Iron Pyrite, Jadeite, Jasper, Kunzite, Magnetite, Pink Tourmaline, Orange Spinel, Spinel, Topaz.

> **Sun in Taurus:** *Birthstone:* Emerald. *Abundance Crystal:* Peridot. *Ritual Crystal:* Boji Stone. *Companion Crystals:* Aquamarine, Aragonite, Azurite, Black Spinel, Blue Chalcedony, Blue Lace Agate, Boji Stone, Botswana Agate, Diamond, Kunzite, Kyanite, Lapis Lazuli, Malachite, Peridot, Rhodonite, Rose Quartz, Rutilated Quartz, Sapphire, Selenite, Tiger's Eye, Topaz, Tourmaline, Variscite.

> **Sun in Gemini:** *Birthstones:* Agate, Tourmaline.

Abundance Crystal: Dendritic Agate. *Ritual Crystal:* Apophyllite. *Companion Crystals:* Apatite, Apophyllite, Aquamarine, Blue Spinel, Calcite, Chrysocolla, Chrysoprase, Citrine, Dendritic Agate, Dendritic Chalcedony, Green Obsidian, Green Tourmaline, Hiddenite, Howlite, Sapphire, Serpentine, Sugilite, Tiger's Eye, Topaz, Tourmalinated and Rutilated Quartz, Variscite.

Sun in Cancer: *Birthstone:* Moonstone. *Abundance Crystal:* Moonstone. *Ritual Crystal:* Calcite. *Companion Crystals:* Amber, Beryl, Brown Spinel, Calcite, Carnelian, Chalcedony, Chrysoprase, Emerald, Howlite, Jasper, Opal, Petalite, Pink Tourmaline, Rhodonite, Ruby.

Sun in Leo: *Birthstone:* Cat or Tiger's Eye. *Abundance Crystal:* Tiger's Eye. *Ritual Crystal:* Red Garnet. *Companion Crystals:* Amber, Boji Stone, Carnelian, Chrysocolla, Citrine, Danburite, Emerald, Garnet, Golden Beryl, Green and Pink Tourmaline, Kunzite, Larimar, Muscovite, Onyx, Orange Calcite, Petalite, Pink Beryl, Pyrolusite, Quartz, Red Obsidian, Rhodochrosite, Ruby, Sunstone, Topaz, Turquoise, Yellow Spinel.

Sun in Virgo: *Birthstones:* Peridot, Sardonyx. *Abundance Crystal:* Moss Agate. *Ritual Crystal:* Moss Agate. *Companion Crystals:* Agate, Amazonite, Amber, Blue Topaz, Carnelian, Cerussite, Chrysocolla, Citrine, Dioptase, Garnet, Magnetite, Moonstone, Moss Agate, Opal, Purple Obsidian, Rubellite, Rutilated Quartz,

Sapphire, Smithsonite, Sodalite, Sugilite, Vanadinite, Violet Spinel, Watermelon Tourmaline.

Sun in Libra: *Birthstones:* Opal, Sapphire. *Abundance Crystal:* Sapphire. *Ritual Crystal:* Apophyllite. *Companion Crystals:* Ametrine, Apophyllite, Aquamarine, Aventurine, Bloodstone, Chiastolite, Chrysolite, Emerald, Green Spinel, Green Tourmaline, Jade, Kunzite, Lapis Lazuli, Lepidolite, Mahogany Obsidian, Moonstone, Peridot, Soulmate, Topaz.

Sun in Scorpio: *Birthstones:* Malachite, Turquoise. *Abundance Crystal:* Hawk Eye. *Ritual Crystal:* Malachite. *Companion Crystals:* Apache Tear, Aquamarine, Beryl, Boji Stone, Charoite, Dioptase, Emerald, Garnet, Green Tourmaline, Herkimer Diamond, Hiddenite, Kunzite, Moonstone, Obsidian, Red Spinel, Rhodochrosite, Ruby, Sceptre Quartz, Smoky Quartz, Topaz, Variscite.

Sun in Sagittarius: *Birthstones:* Topaz, Turquoise. *Abundance Crystal:* Citrine. *Ritual Crystal:* Red Spinel. *Companion Crystals:* Amethyst, Azurite, Blue Lace Agate, Chalcedony, Charoite, Citrine, Dark Blue Spinel, Dioptase, Garnet, Gold Sheen Obsidian, Iolite with Sunstone, Labradorite, Lapis Lazuli, Malachite, Pink Tourmaline, Rhyolite, Ruby, Smoky Quartz, Snowflake Obsidian, Sodalite, Spinel, Wulfenite.

Sun in Capricorn: *Birthstones:* Garnet, Onyx. *Abundance Crystal:* Ruby. *Ritual Crystal:* Reddish-brown Aragonite. *Companion Crystals:* Amber,

Aragonite, Azurite, Carnelian, Fluorite, Galena, Green and Black Tourmaline, Jet, Labradorite, Magnetite, Malachite, Obsidian, Peridot, Quartz, Ruby, Serpentine, Smoky Quartz, Snowflake Obsidian, Stibnite, Turquoise.

Sun in Aquarius: *Birthstone:* Aquamarine. *Abundance Crystal:* Quartz. *Ritual Crystal:* Angelite. *Companion Crystals:* Amber, Amethyst, Angelite, Atacamite, Blue Celestite, Blue Obsidian, Boji Stone, Chrysoprase, Fluorite, Fuchsite, Labradorite, Magnetite, Moonstone.

Sun in Pisces: *Birthstones:* Amethyst. *Abundance Crystal:* Bloodstone. *Ritual Crystal:* Blue Lace Agate. *Companion Crystals:* Aquamarine, Beryl, Bloodstone, Blue Lace Agate, Calcite, Chrysoprase, Fluorite, Labradorite, Moonstone, Selenite, Smithsonite, Turquoise.

– Lunar crystals –

Lunar crystals: Blue Moonstone, Celtic White Chevron Quartz, Moonstone, Pearl, Petalite, Rainbow Moonstone, Rhomboid Selenite, Selenite, Snow Quartz, White/Clear Calcite

Moon in Aries: Snow Quartz/Celtic White Chevron. *Intuition Crystal:* Ametrine. *Companion Crystals:* Aragonite, Aventurine, Bloodstone, Blue Lace Agate, Carnelian, Cerussite, Chrysoberyl, Chrysoprase, Hawk's Eye, Iron Pyrite, Jasper, Kunzite, Magnesite, Red Jade, Rhodonite, Ruby, Sunstone.

Moon in Taurus: Rutilated Quartz. *Intuition Crystal:* Selenite. *Companion Crystals:* Apache Tear, Beryl, Blue Tourmaline, Green Agate, Green Calcite, Idocrase, Kunzite, Kyanite, Lepidolite, Magnetite, Malachite, Mookaite, Peridot, Prehnite, Rhodonite, Sunstone.

Moon in Gemini: Apophyllite. *Intuition Crystal:* Aqua Aura. *Companion Crystals:* Aquamarine, Aventurine, Blue Selenite, Blue Topaz, Blue Tourmaline, Calcite, Carnelian, Charoite, Kyanite, Rhodochrosite, Rhomboid Blue Calcite, Ruby, Sapphire, Snowflake Obsidian, Sugilite, Variscite.

Moon in Cancer: Moonstone/Black Moonstone. *Intuition Crystal:* Blue Moonstone. *Companion Crystals:* Carnelian, Chalcedony, Chrysocolla, Chrysoprase, Dioptase, Howlite, Jade, Jasper, Moonstone, Morganite, Opal, Pearl, Petalite, Pink Tourmaline, Rhodonite, Selenite, Sodalite, Sunstone.

Moon in Leo: Golden Healer. *Intuition Crystal:* Yellow Calcite. *Companion Crystals:* Ametrine, Apophyllite, Aventurine, Brown Opal, Calcite, Carnelian, Chrysocolla, Citrine, Dioptase, Fuchsite, Kunzite, Larimar, Morganite, Rhodochrosite, Rose Quartz, Tiger's Eye, Topaz.

Moon in Virgo: Selenite. *Intuition Crystal:* Kyanite. *Companion Crystals:* Amethyst, Azurite, Blue Topaz, Carnelian, Charoite, Chrysoberyl, Citrine, Fuchsite, Garnet, Hiddenite, Jasper, Peridot, Pietersite, Sardonyx, Smoky Quartz, Staurolite.

Moon in Libra: Rose Quartz. *Intuition Crystal:* Opal.

Companion Crystals: Amethyst, Aquamarine, Blue Topaz, Calcite, Celestite, Chrysoberyl, Iolite, Jade, Larimar, Mangano Calcite, Rhodochrosite, Sardonyx, Sugilite, Watermelon Tourmaline, Wulfenite.

Moon in Scorpio: Smoky Quartz. *Intuition Crystal:* Herkimer Diamond. *Companion Crystals:* Agate, Apache Tear, Beryl, Black Obsidian, Charoite, Dioptase, Green Jasper, Hawk's Eye, Herkimer Diamond, Labradorite, Malachite, Rhodochrosite, Rhodonite, Rutilated Quartz, Sceptre Quartz, Smithsonite, Turquoise.

Moon in Sagittarius: Apophyllite. *Intuition Crystal:* Lapis Lazuli. *Companion Crystals:* Azurite, Bytownite, Cerussite, Charoite, Emerald, Garnet, Lapis Lazuli, Lepidolite, Moss Agate, Nebula Stone, Okenite, Rhodochrosite, Rhyolite, Sodalite, Topaz, Wulfenite.

Moon in Capricorn: Snow Quartz. *Intuition Crystal:* Phantom Quartz. *Companion Crystals:* Ametrine, Aquamarine, Blue Lace Agate, Calcite, Charoite, Chrysanthemum Stone, Galena, Garnet, Iron Pyrite, Magnesite, Moonstone, Pietersite, Pyrolusite, Rhodochrosite, Serpentine.

Moon in Aquarius: Clear Quartz. *Intuition Crystal:* Aquamarine. *Companion Crystals:* Aquamarine, Beryl, Boji Stones, Celestite, Cerussite, Chalcedony, Charoite, Chiastolite, Chrysoprase, Gold Sheen Obsidian, Moldavite, Rhodonite, Rose Quartz, Selenite, Soulmate Crystal, Sulphur in Quartz, Vanadinite.

Moon in Pisces: Amethyst. *Intuition Crystal:* Celestite. *Companion Crystals:* Angelite, Aventurine, Blue Lace Agate, Boji Stones, Celestite, Chiastolite, Chrysoprase, Cymophane, Danburite, Fire Agate, Fluorite, Fuchsite, Jasper, Kunzite, Magnesite, Morganite, Opal Aura Quartz, Rhodochrosite, Ruby in Zoisite, Selenite, Sunstone, Tiger's Eye.

– Planetary crystals –

Chiron: Charoite, Grape Chalcedony

Jupiter: Amethyst, Azurite, Cassiterite, Chalcedony, Chrysocolla, Citrine, Diamond, Emerald, Grape Chalcedony, Heliodor, Iris Quartz, Jasper, Lapis Lazuli, Malachite, Sugilite, Topaz, Turquoise, Yellow Apatite, Yellow Sapphire, White Topaz, Zircon, and tin-bearing stones

Mars: Agate, Amethyst, Beryl, Bixbite, Bloodstone, Bronzite, Carnelian, Cinnabar (*caution: toxic*), Citrine, Coral", Garnet, Heliodor, Hematite, Magnetite (Lodestone), Mookaite Jasper, Pyrite, Quartz, Red Jasper, Ruby, Sardonyx, Tiger's Eye, Topaz, Triplite, Zircon and iron-bearing stones

Mercury: Agate, Amber, Aquamarine, Auralite 23, Aventurine, Black Moonstone, Blue Lace Agate, Blue Topaz, Calcite, Chalcedony, Chrysoprase, Cinnabar (*caution: toxic*), Citrine, Cymophane, Diopside, Emerald, Fire Agate, Fluorite, Green Jade, Green Tourmaline, Hematite, Jasper, Lapis Lace, Moldavite, Peridot, Pyrite, Rhodochrosite, Sapphire, Sodalite, Tiger's Eye, Tsavorite

Garnet, Turquoise and silver-bearing crystals

Neptune: Amethyst, Andara Glass, Aquamarine, Blue Calcite, Bytownite, Celestite, Coral", Covellite, Fluorite, Jade, Kyanite, Labradorite, Lapis Lace, Lapis Lazuli, Larimar, Lemurian Aquatine Calcite, Libyan Glass Tektite, Pearl Sapphire, Rainbow Moonstone, Sea Foam Flint, Sea Sediment Jasper, Selenite, Sugilite and zinc-bearing crystals

North Node: Anandalite™, Auralite 23, Hessonite Garnet, Orange Zircon, Record Keeper Ruby, Spessartine Garnet, Trigonic Quartz, White Agate

In Aries: Aventurine, Garnet, Tiger's Eye *and see Solar and Lunar stones*

In Taurus: Emerald, Fluorite, Malachite and *see Solar and Lunar stones*

In Gemini: Carnelian, Howlite, Moonstone *and see Solar and Lunar stones*

In Cancer: Rainbow Moonstone, Rhodonite, Rose Quartz *and see Solar and Lunar stones*

In Leo: Pyrite, Ruby, Sunstone, Turquoise *and see Solar and Lunar stones*

In Virgo: Agate, Blue Chalcedony, Onyx *and see solar and lunar stones*

In Libra: Andaluscite, Atlantean Lovestar (Candle/Celestial Quartz), Jasper, Mangano Calcite, Prehnite, Rose Quartz *and see Solar and Lunar stones*

In Scorpio: Citrine, Labradorite, Selenite, Smoky Quartz *and see Solar and Lunar stones*

In Sagittarius: Hematite, Lapis Lazuli, Obsidian *and*

see Solar and Lunar stones

In Capricorn: Aragonite, Bloodstone, Iolite in Sunstone, Topaz *and see Solar and Lunar stones*

In Aquarius: Charoite, Moldavite, Watermelon Tourmaline *and see Solar and Lunar stones*

In Pisces: Amethyst, Apophyllite, Sugilite *and see Solar and Lunar stones*

South Node: Ancestralite, Beryl, Cat's Eye, Chrysoberyl, Cymophane, Lakelandite, Tiger's Eye

Pluto: Ancestralite, Black Obsidian, Black Tourmaline, Bumble Bee Jasper, Chalcedony Tears, Fire Agate, Fire Obsidian, Jet, Kunzite, Kyanite, Labradorite, Lakelandite, Moldavite, Ruby, Smoky Elestial Quartz, Smoky Quartz, Snowflake Obsidian, Tourmalinated Quartz, Zincite, and volcanic crystals

Saturn: Agate, Agrellite, Amber, Aquamarine, Azurite, Blue Sapphire, Blue Scapolite, Blue Spinel, Chalcedony, Diamond, Epidote, Galena (*caution: toxic*), Green Calcite, Hematite, Indicolite, Iolite-and-Sunstone, Jet, Lapis Lazuli, Magnetite, Obsidian, Onyx, Pyrite, Sapphire, Sardonyx, Smoky Quartz, Stibnite, Topaz, lead and iron-bearing crystals

South Node: Agate, Ancestralite, Apatite, Black Tourmaline, Chrysotile, Dumortierite, Lakelandite, Lemurian Seed Quartz, Quartz, Trigonic Quartz

Uranus: Aquamarine, Aventurine, Azurite, Blue Topaz, Chalcedony, Labradorite, Lapis Lazuli, Quartz, Rutilated Quartz, Sapphire, Tourmalinated Quartz, and uranium-bearing crystals (*caution: radioactive*)

Venus: Alabaster, Amazonite, Beryl, Carnelian, Chrysocolla, Chrysoprase, Cobalto Calcite, Copper-coloured Pyrite, Coral", Diamond, Emerald, Green Aventurine, Jasper, Kunzite, Lapis Lazuli, Larimar, Malachite, Mangano Calcite, Marcasite, Peridot, Quartz, Rhodochrosite, Rose Quartz, Roselite, Ruby, Sapphire, Sphalerite, Tourmaline, Turquoise, Zircon and copper-bearing crystals

– Astrological body-crystal correspondences –

Sun: *Heart:* Green Aventurine, Mangano Calcite, Rhodochrosite, Rhodonite, Rose Quartz, Tugtupite. *Back/spinal column:* Fluorite, Magnesite. *Thymus:* Amethyst, Bloodstone, Citrine, Quantum Quattro, Que Sera, Smithsonite. *Paternal issues* see page 259.

Moon: *Breasts/body fluids:* Moonstone, Selenite. *Reproductive system:* Carnelian, Smoky Quartz. *Bile duct:* Emerald, Gaspeite, Red Jasper. *Digestive system:* Amethyst, Chrysocolla, Green Jasper. *Liver:* Bloodstone, Carnelian, Yellow Fluorite, Yellow Jasper. *Pancreas:* Amber, Bloodstone, Green Calcite, Lapis Lace, Red Serpentine. *Maternal issues/heredity* see page 259.

Chiron: *Immune system:* Bloodstone, Quantum Quattro, Que Sera. *Thighs:* Charoite, Smoky Quartz. *Genitals:* Menalite, Red Jasper.

Mars: *Muscles:* Hematite, Magnesite, Rhodonite. *Urogenitals:* Blue Aventurine, Kyanite. *Will-assertion-aggression issues* see page 95.

Mercury: *Respiration:* Amber, Charoite, Fluorite. *Brain:*

Banded Agate, Kyanite, Labradorite. *Nervous system:* Blue Lace Agate, Green Jade. *Communication issues and over-thinking* see pages 214 and 288.

Jupiter: *Liver:* Amethyst, Bloodstone, Gaspeite, Yellow Jasper. *Pituitary gland:* Iolite, Sapphire. *Overindulgence* see page 186.

Neptune: *Nervous system:* Banded Agate, Blue Lace Agate, Green Jade, Lapis Lace. *Hypothalamus:* Blue Lace Agate. *Psychic abilities* see page 199.

Saturn: *Bones:* Fluorite, Magnetite. *Gall bladder:* Amber, Citrine, Gaspeite, Malachite. *Spleen:* Amber, Bloodstone. *Skin:* Agate, Jasper. *Teeth:* Fluorite. Karmic issues, repressions and denial.

Uranus: *Circulatory system:* Hematite, Ruby. *Pineal gland:* Amethyst, Moonstone. *Chemical-electrical circuitry in brain:* Banded Agate, Kyanite.

Venus: *Throat:* Blue Lace Agate, Turquoise. *Kidneys:* Bloodstone, Fluorite, Jade. *Lumbar region:* Carnelian. *Veins:* Rhodochrosite, Smithsonite. *Parathyroid:* Kyanite, Malachite.

Pluto: *Reproductive system:* Carnelian, Jasper, Malachite, Smoky Quartz. *Power issues* see page 259.

– Elemental crystals –

Air: *Antidotes to weak Air:* Aquamarine and light blue stones such as Blue Chalcedony, Blue Fluorite, Blue Lace Agate, Lapis Lace, Turquoise. *Antidotes to excess Air:* deep blue and violet colours; Aquamarine, Azurite, Black Moonstone, Blue Topaz, Blue Tourmaline,

Chrysocolla, Green Calcite, Green Fluorite, Lapis Lace, Lapis Lazuli, Sapphire, Sodalite.

Earth: *Antidotes to weak Earth:* brown stones such as Ancestralite, Flint, Picture Jasper, Tiger Iron or Tiger's Eye. *Antidotes to excess Earth:* Anandalite, Selenite, Smoky Quartz, light yellow stones such as Citrine or Grey Labradorite.

Fire: *Antidotes to weak Fire:* Bloodstone, Carnelian, Fire Agate, Garnet, Orange Calcite, Red Jasper, Ruby, Sunstone, Topaz. *Antidotes to excess Fire:* Aquamarine, Aventurine, Emerald, Green Calcite, Green Garnet, Malachite.

Water: *Antidotes to weak Water:* Aquamarine, Blue Flint, Hematite, Moss Agate, Muscovite, Opal, Pearl, Smoky Elestial Quartz, Tourmaline. *Antidotes to excess Water:* Fluorite, Green Aventurine, Kunzite, Pink Tourmaline, Rose Quartz. If ungrounded and boundary-less, Healer's Gold, Hematite, Labradorite, Mohawkite, Smoky Quartz.

Note: For further information see The Astrology Bible *and* The Crystal Zodiac. *To calculate your birthchart see www.astro.com/cgi/ade.cgi.*

– Additional astro-information –

Challenging aspects, transmuting a pattern: Ancestralite, Auralite 23, Blue Kyanite, Brandenberg Amethyst, Chrysocolla, Cradle of Life (Humanity), Eye of the Storm, Fluorite, Freedom Stone, Herkimer Diamond, Jade, Quartz, Rhodozite, Trigonic Quartz and crystals for the planets involved.

Days of the week:
Sunday: Diamond, Pear, Sunstone, Topaz
Monday: Emerald, Moonstone, Pearl
Tuesday: Emerald, Ruby, Star Sapphire, Topaz
Wednesday: Amethyst, Magnetite, Star Ruby, Turquoise
Thursday: Carnelian, Cat's Eye, Sapphire
Friday: Alexandrite, Cat's Eye, Emerald, Ruby
Saturday: Amethyst, Diamond, Labradorite, Turquoise

Fixed Stars and star systems: Etched Quartz, Lightbraries, Lightning-struck Quartz, Starbrary Amethyst, Starbrary Quartz, Starseed Quartz, Stellar Beam Calcite.

'Return home'/contact star beings: Ajo Blue Calcite, Apophyllite, Cerussite, Galaxyite, Glaucophane, Infinite Stone, Labradorite, Lazurite, Lemurian Seed, Libyan Glass Tektite, Moldavite, Mount Shasta Opal, Nebula Stone, Record Keeper Quartz, Scolecite, Star Hollandite, Starbrary Quartz, Starseed Quartz, Stellar Beam Calcite, Sugarblade Quartz, Tektite, Trigonic

Specific Starbrary Quartz Crystals star system connections:

Andromeda: Almost always double terminated. The keys may be tiny. The sides appear to be layered, but with no raised face termination. It's as if the ET crystals overgrew the main one. These appear to be connected to crystals from Cassiopeia and the Pleiadian peoples.

Cassiopeia: Flowing lines and symbols along the sides of the crystal. May exhibit key markings.

Leo: Linear patterns on sides.

Orion: Titanium included quartz with the deep ridges and furrows that create definite glyphs in the faces of the crystal rather than the sides.

Pleiades: Geometric symbols (triangles, squares, circles, etc.) along the sides, often with profound keys.

Ursa Minor: Indented triangles and dashes – a kind of Morse Code – resembling a meteor shower.

Star and star system connections:

Aldebaran: Garnet, Grape Chalcedony, Ruby

Algol: Diamond

Algorab: Black Onyx

Alphecca: Golden Topaz

Andromeda: Pearl

Antares: Amethyst, Sardonyx

Arcturus: Blue Apatite, Green Jasper

Capella: Blue Sapphire

Deneb Algedi: Blue Chalcedony

Pleiades: Celestite, K2, Lemurian Seed, Moldavite, Quartz (Rock Crystal), Starbrary Quartz

Polaris: Magnetite

Pole Star: Hematite, Magnetite

Procyon: Banded Agate

Regulus: Garnet, Granite

Sirius: Bery

Spica: Emerald, Jasper
Vega: Howlite, Peridot (Chrysolite)

Gems of Spring: Amethyst, Chrysoberyl, Diamond, Emerald, Peridot, Pink Topaz, Spinel, Rubellite
Gems of Summer: Alexandrite, Fire Opal, Garnet, Pink Topaz, Ruby, Spinel
Gems of Autumn: Cairngorm (Smoky Citrine), Peridot, Quartz, Sapphire, Topaz, Tourmaline, Zircon
Gems of Winter: Diamond, Labradorite, Moonstone, Pearl, Quartz, Turquoise, White Sapphire

Hours of the Day (from sunrise)

1 Zircon
2 Emerald
3 Beryl
4 Topaz
5 Ruby
6 Opal
7 Peridot
8 Amethyst
9 Kunzite
10 Sapphire
11 Garnet
12 Diamond

Hours of the Night (from sunset)

1 Morion Quartz
2 Hematite

3   Malachite
4   Lapis Lazuli
5   Turquoise
6   Tourmaline
7   Sardonyx
8   Chalcedony
9   Jade
10 Jasper
11 Lodestone
12 Onyx

Months of the year: Talismanic gems[6]

January: Garnet, Serpentine, Zircon
February: Amethyst, Pearl, Zircon
March: Bloodstone, Jasper
April: Diamond, Sapphire
May: Agate, Carnelian, Chalcedony, Emerald
June: Agate, Cat's Eye, Chalcedony, Emerald, Pearl, Turquoise
July: Carnelian, Onyx, Ruby, Sardonyx, Turquoise
August: Alexandrite, Carnelian, Moonstone, Ruby, Sardonyx, Topaz
September: Peridot, Sapphire, Sardonyx, Zircon
October: Aquamarine, Beryl, Coral", Opal, Tourmaline
November: Cat's Eye, Pearl, Topaz
December: Bloodstone, Chrysoprase, Lapis Lazuli, Ruby, Turquoise

  "Always use ethically sourced Coral.

Part VI: Specific crystal essences with A-Z Directories

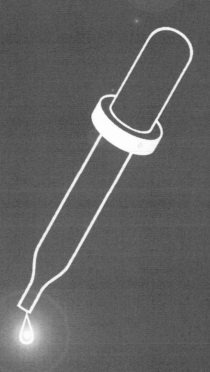

Abundance and Aspirational

essences

Select 1–4 crystals when creating your essence.

Abundance is a state of mind that encompasses prosperity and so much more. Our attitude to prosperity determines how much abundance we enjoy and whether we live a fundamentally satisfied and enriched life. Prosperity consciousness is about feeling satisfied and secure with what you have, living an enriching and fulfilling life, sharing life's bounty, feeling gratitude and trusting that the universe provides appropriately for your needs. Poverty consciousness, on the other hand, is about always feeling a lack and is a base chakra security issue.

Steps to abundance

- Change your mental program: what your mind conceives, it achieves.
- Set realistic goals but don't be afraid to dream and aim high.
- Measure your self-worth by who you are, not what you do or what you have.
- Follow your bliss: do what you love and abundance follows.
- Obey the fundamental law of attraction: like

follows like.

- Believe you can fulfil your dreams.
- Gratitude: notice and appreciate all the small joys of everyday life.
- Recognise that the universe wants you to succeed.
- Focus on exactly what you want to attract right now.
- Give yourself time, kindness and compassion.
- Avoid doubt and guilt and no longer procrastinate.
- Let go of fear or self-pity.
- Share what you have and take pleasure in giving.
- Balance your earth star, base and sacral chakras.

Essences can be created using the prescriptions in the A-Z Directory below and the power of astral-magic can be harnessed by adding crystals appropriate to the hour, day, week or month to the mix.

A-Z Directory

– A –

Achievable dream or illusion? Distinguish between: Carnelian, Purple Tourmaline

Attracting money: Carnelian, Citrine, Garnet, Green Grossular Garnet, Jet, Manifestation Quartz, Quartz Generator, Yellow Sapphire

– B –

Budgeting: Cinnabar, Citrine, Green Spinel, Hematite, Peridot

– C –

Cosmic ordering: Green Aventurine, Green Calcite, Iron Pyrite, Quartz, Topaz

Creative success: Andradite Garnet, Aventurine, Dendritic Agate, Garnet, Iolite-Sunstone, Lapis Lazuli, Manifestation Quartz, Quartz Generator, Tiger's Eye

> **bringing dreams into being:** Black Moonstone, Calcite, Carnelian, Flint, Hematite, Heulandite, Iron Pyrite, Jade, Manifestation Quartz, Quartz Generator, Red Chalcedony, Ruby, Smoky Quartz

– D –

Driving test: Carnelian, Fluorite, Grape Chalcedony, Red Jasper, Tourmalinated Quartz

– F –

Feeling positive: Carnelian, Iron Pyrite, Pinolith, Red Jasper

Finding the right job: Black or Dark Blue Sapphire, Cinnabar, Citrine, Golden Tiger's Eye, Holey Stones, Iron Pyrite, Jet, Magnetite, Manifestation Quartz, Moss Agate, Plume Agate, Quartz Generator, Tiger's Eye, Tree or other Agate

– G –

Gratitude: Apatite, Green Apatite, Green Aventurine, Hiddenite, Larimar, Pietersite, Pink Sapphire, Rose Quartz, Selenite, Sodalite, Tiger's Eye

– I –

Inner peace: Amethyst, Ammonite, Calcite, Chrysoprase, Eye of the Storm (Judy's Jasper), Grape Chalcedony, Jade, Prairie Tanzanite, Rose Quartz, Uvarovite Garnet

– J –

Joy bringers: Cavansite, Chrysoprase, Citrine, Emerald, Green Tourmaline, Mangano Calcite, Orange or Yellow Jade, Pink Chalcedony, Poppy Jasper, Red Calcite, Ruby in Kyanite or Zoisite, Sapphire, Stellar Beam Calcite, Sunstone, Topaz Orange or Yellow or Golden Calcite

– L –

Life purpose: Long flat Quartz with one absolutely smooth side. Brandenberg Amethyst, Cradle of Life

(Humankind), Herkimer Diamond, Lapis Lazuli, Moldavite

– M –

Manifestation, remove block to: Calcite, Chlorite Quartz, Malachite, Manifestation Quartz, Obsidian, Rose Quartz, Selenite, Smoky Quartz. *Chakra:* solar plexus, heart, Gaia gateway

Material success: Carnelian, Cinnabar, Citrine, Jet, Manifestation Quartz, Morganite, Quartz Generator, Spinel, square-cut Garnets, Tree Agate

– N –

New beginnings: Iron Pyrite, Moonstone, White Calcite. *Timing: new moon.*

– O –

Optimism: Carnelian, Citrine, Red Jasper, Topaz

– P –

Persistence: Adamite, Agate, Flint, Hematite, Moss Agate, Onyx, self-healed crystals, Snowflake Obsidian

Poverty consciousness, reverse: Citrine, Green Calcite, Peridot. *Chakra:* base

Prosperity: Ammolite, Carnelian, Citrine, Goldstone, Green Aventurine, Jade, Tiger's Eye, Turquoise, Yellow Sapphire

– S –

Sensible spending: Green Quartz (Prasiolite), Green Tourmaline, Hematite, Jet and Peridot

Succeeding in your goals: Citrine, Hemimorphite, Manifestation Quartz, Quartz Generator, Red Chalcedony, Ruby, Tiger's Eye, Topaz, Turquoise

– T –

Trust: Calcite, Kunzite, Lavender Jade, Peridot, Prehnite, Rose Quartz, Rubellite (Pink Tourmaline)

– W –

Work-leisure balance: Agate, Almandine Garnet, Andradite Garnet, Aventurine, bicoloured crystals, Calcite, Grape Chalcedony, Lavender Jade, Merlinite, Prairie Tanzanite, Turquoise

Writing: Calligraphy Stone, Chinese Writing Stone, Lapis Lazuli (develop 'bat ears'), Pink Chalcedony, Triplite

Addictions and underlying issues essences

Many addictions have at their base an underlying sense of lack, of something missing from life. A lack of meaning, for instance. Or a black hole of spiritual loneliness. As someone once said, "It's a search for spirit in the wrong bottle." Such a lack can be addressed through crystals for expanding consciousness (see page 197) and by placing an essence to awaken the higher chakras. Addiction can also arise from prescribed medication, in which case an essence may be required to assist with pain (see page 190) or withdrawal symptoms. Addiction may also be self-medication for allergies, bipolar and other mental or physiological disturbances. In many cases the underlying physiological or psychological issues will need to be addressed in addition to the physical addiction and withdrawal symptoms.

Addictions may arise from karmic causes (see page 242) or be passed down the family line (see ancestral healing page 247), and these issues will need to be addressed first. If you have a serious alcohol or drug addiction problem, please seek the advice of your doctor or a drug rehab clinic when detoxing. Crystal essences can support your recovery process and assist in dulling down cravings.

Where a left and a right-hand crystal is indicated create two crystal essences, one from each crystal, and rub the essences into the palms of the appropriate hands at the same time. This has been anecdotally proven to be more effective than combining the two crystals into one essence.

Some of the crystal combinations in this directory arise from the pioneering work of Donna Cunningham (see Resources).

A-Z Addictions Directory

Choose 1–4 crystals from the substance list when creating your essence. Crystals for different issues can be combined as appropriate or used for concatenation (see page 70).

Note: If you have an alcohol or heroin addiction, use alternative preservation methods rather than alcohol for the mother tincture and further dilutions.

– A –

Alcohol: Amethyst, Celestite, Danburite, Dioptase, Iolite, Labradorite, Quartz, Tiger's Eye. *Chakra*: base, sacral, solar plexus, crown. Or: Citrine (*rub on left palm*) and Celestite (*rub on right palm*). *Chakra*: base, sacral, navel, heart. *Or disperse around the aura. And see Cravings. Note: do not use alcohol as a preservative (see page 62).*

Amphetamines: Lepidolite, Ruby, Selenite and grounding crystals (see page 266). *Chakra:* alta major

– B –

Bipolar disorder: Bastnasite, Brucite, Halite, Kunzite, Lepidocrosite, Lepidolite, Lithium Quartz, Montebrasite, Tantalite. *Chakra:* base and third eye, alta major

– C –

Caffeine: Green Tourmaline, Malachite, Peridot, Quartz, Rooster Tail Quartz. *Chakra:* solar plexus, base, sacral, navel, heart. *Or disperse around the aura. And see Cravings.*

Chocolate: Amethyst, Citrine, Jasper

Cocaine: Dioptase, Fluorite, Green Aventurine, Labradorite, Selenite. Aventurine (*rub on right palm*) and Selenite (*rub on left palm*). *Chakra:* base, sacral, navel, heart, alta major. *Or disperse around aura and head, and inhale essence. And see Cravings.*

Codependency: Amethyst Aura Quartz, Bytownite, Dumortierite, Fenster Quartz, Iolite, Quantum Quattro, Rose Quartz, Sichuan Quartz, Vera Cruz Amethyst, Zenotine. *Chakra:* base, dantien, causal vortex

Compassion for oneself and others: Ajoite, Brandenberg Amethyst, Cobalto Calcite, Erythrite, Gaia Stone, Geothite, Golden Healer, Green Diopside, Green Ridge Quartz, Greenlandite, Mangano Vesuvianite, Paraiba Tourmaline, Rhodolite Garnet, Shaman Quartz, Smoky Cathedral Quartz, Starseed Quartz, Tangerose, Tanzanite, Tugtupite. *Chakra:* heart seed

Compulsive or obsessive thoughts: Ammolite, Auralite 23, Azurite, Barite, Bytownite, K2, Optical Calcite, Rhomboid Selenite, Scolecite, Spirit Quartz, Tantalite. *Chakra:* third eye, crown

Cravings, obsessions: Amber, Amethyst, Black Tourmaline, Blue Topaz, Carnelian, Citrine, Diamond, Fire Agate, Galena, Garnet, Hematite, Iolite, Kiwi Stone (Sesame Jasper), Labradorite, Lepidolite, Peridot, Quartz, Rhyolite, Rose Quartz, Ruby, Tiger's Eye. *Chakra:* base, sacral, dantien, navel, past life, causal vortex

– D –

Depression: Ajo Blue Calcite, Amethyst, Clinohumite, Dianite, Eisenkiesel, Eudialyte, Flint, Kunzite, Lepidolite, Macedonian Opal, Maw Sit Sit, Montebrasite, Orange Kyanite, Pink Sunstone, Porphyrite (Chinese Letter Stone), Rainbow Geothite, Sillimanite, Spiders Web Obsidian, Sunstone, Tugtupite. *Chakra:* solar plexus

Depressive psychosis: Kunzite, Lithium Quartz, Tugtupite. *Chakra:* higher heart (treat under the supervision of a qualified crystal healer)

Despair: Novaculite, Pyrite in Quartz, Vera Cruz Amethyst. *Chakra*: heart

Despondency: Purpurite. *Chakra:* heart

Determination: Hematite, Picture Jasper, Rhyolite, Tiger Iron *and see Willpower page 192*

– E –

Eating disorders: *see Bulimia (page 306), Anorexia (page 305), Body dysmorphia (page 306)*

– F –

Food, binge and comfort eating: Amethyst, Apatite, Carnelian, Polychrome Jasper, Sunstone. *Chakra:* base, sacral, navel, solar plexus. *And see Cravings.*

– G –

Gambling: Amethyst, Chrysoprase, Clear Quartz, Green Aventurine, Iolite, Rose Quartz. *Chakra:* base, sacral, navel, solar plexus. *And see Cravings.*

– H –

Heroin: Amethyst Elestial, Aventurine, Blue Moonstone, Brandenberg Amethyst, Dioptase, Eudialyte, Fluorite, Lepidolite, Rhyolite, Rose Quartz, Spirit Quartz, Trigonic Quartz, Vera Cruz Amethyst. Selenite (*rub on right palm*) and Aventurine (*rub on left palm*). *Chakra:* base, sacral, navel, heart. *And see Cravings. Note: Do not use alcohol as a preservative as the brain receptors sensitive to heroin also fit alcohol molecules (see page 62).*

– I –

'Identified patient'/takes on the family pain or disease: Dioptase, Fenster Quartz, Gaia's Blood Flint, Grape Chalcedony, Green Zoisite, Mangano Calcite, Pinolith, Polychrome Jasper, Thulite. *Chakra:* navel

Investing without undue risk: Goldstone, Malachite, Peridot, Prehnite

– L –

Liver, detoxify: Amechlorite, Bastnasite, Biotite, Chlorite Quartz, Eye of the Storm, Gaspeite, Iolite, Kambaba Jasper, Klinoptilolith, Larvikite, Lepidolite, Malachite, Mtrolite, Pyrite in Magnesite, Rainbow Covellite, Richterite, Seraphinite, Shungite, Smoky Quartz with Aegerine, Thunder Egg

– M –

Marijuana: Azurite, Dioptase, Herderite, Quartz. Carnelian (*rub on left palm*) and Azurite (*rub on right*

palm). *Chakra:* base, sacral, navel, heart, alta major. *Or disperse essence around the head. And see Cravings.*

– N –

Negative self-image: Carnelian, Citrine, Golden Calcite, Lepidolite, Rose Quartz, Sodalite. *Chakra:* heart.

Nicotine: Botswana Agate, Dioptase, Peridot, Quartz. Smoky Quartz (*rub on right palm*) and Blue Fluorite (*rub on left palm*). *Chakra:* base, sacral, navel, heart, alta major. *Or disperse essence around the head. And see Cravings.*

– O –

Obesity: Black Onyx, Diamond, Moonstone, Polychrome Jasper, Tourmaline, Zircon. *Chakra:* navel *and see Weight page 192*

– P –

Pain: Azurite, Bastnasite, Bird's Eye Jasper, Blue Euclase, Bronzite, Cathedral Quartz, Eilat Stone, Flint, Hungarian Quartz, Khutnohorite, Lapis Lazuli, Quantum Quattro, Reinerite, Rhodozite, Stichtite and Serpentine, Wind Fossil Agate. *Rub over site.*

Pain relief: see Stress and PTSD page 286

Painful feelings, assimilate: Khutnohorite, Mangano Calcite, Pinolith, Rhodolite Garnet, Tugtupite. *Chakra:* heart

Panic attack: see Stress and PTSD page 286

Paracetamol and pain-killers: Apophyllite, Azurite, Cathedral Quartz, Lapis Lazuli, Polychrome Jasper,

Rhomboid Selenite. *Chakra:* third eye. *Or disperse essence around the head. And see Cravings.*

'Poor me' syndrome/victim mentality/Karpman dramas: Chrome Dioptase, Green Zoisite, Lemurian Jade, Rhodochrosite, Rose Quartz, Sugilite, Thulite. *Chakra:* solar plexus and heart

– S –

Saviour/rescuer complex: Cassiterite, Chrome Diopside, Sugilite, Thulite

Self-acceptance: Lavender Quartz, Lemurian Seed, Orange Phantom, Peach Selenite, Quantum Quattro, Tangerose, Tugtupite. *Chakra:* heart, higher heart

Self-confidence: Blue Quartz, Lemurian Seed, Nunderite, Pink Sunstone. *Chakra:* solar plexus

Self-defeating programs, overcome: Desert Rose, Drusy Quartz, Kinoite, Nuummite, Paraiba Tourmaline, Quantum Quattro, Strawberry Quartz

Self-discipline: Blue Quartz, Dumortierite, Scapolite, Sillimanite

Self-esteem: Eisenkiesel, Graphic Smoky Quartz (Zebra Stone), Hackmanite, Lazulite, Morion, Nzuri Moyo, Pink Phantom, Strawberry Quartz, Tinguaite. *Chakra:* base, sacral, dantien, heart, higher heart

Self-forgiveness: Chinese Red Quartz, Eudialyte, Mangano Calcite, Pink Crackle Quartz, Rose Quartz, Spirit Quartz, Steatite, Tugtupite. *Chakra:* heart

Self-hatred (combating): Blizzard Stone, Mangano Calcite, Quantum Quattro, Tugtupite. *Chakra:* base

Self-sabotaging behaviour, overcome: Agrellite, Quantum Quattro, Scapolite

Sex: Agate, Amethyst, Garnet, Grape Chalcedony, Green Aventurine, Prairie Tanzanite, Rhodonite, Rose Quartz. *Chakra:* earth star, base, sacral, dantien, navel. *Or disperse on pillow. And see Cravings.*

Smoking: see Nicotine

Sugar and sweeteners: Grape Chalcedony, Prairie Tanzanite, Quartz, Smoky Quartz. Rose Quartz (*rub on left palm*) and Clear Quartz (*rub on right palm*). *Chakra:* earth star, base, sacral, dantien, navel. *Or disperse around the aura or on to the heart and higher heart chakras. And see Cravings.*

– W –

Weight control: Amethyst, Angelite, Apatite, Bloodstone, Blue Apatite, Carnelian, Rose Quartz, Unakite

Weight due to overeating: Green Tourmaline, Kyanite, Polychrome Jasper, Seraphinite and see Food above

Weight loss: Bloodstone, Green Tourmaline, Iolite, Prehnite, Seraphinite, Unakite

Weight, under-eating: Danburite, Eye of the Storm, Grape Chalcedony, Mangano Calcite, Polychrome Jasper, Rose Quartz, Unakite *and see Anorexia and Body dysmorphia, pages 305 and 306*

Willpower: Garnet, Hematite, Pyrite, Red Jasper, Rhodonite, Rhyolite, Tiger Iron, Tiger's Eye, Yellow Jasper, Yellow Sapphire

Consciousness expanding and journeying essences

Expansion of consciousness and multidimensional exploration is activated mainly through opening the higher chakras such as the soul star, stellar gateway and the causal vortex (see pages 101–102) and removing blockages that literally allow you to open your mind. Expanded consciousness also encompasses the angelic realm. Choose crystals from their associated colour or connection for angelic essence-creation. Always remember to ground yourself when taking consciousness expanding essences and close-down the higher chakras afterwards.

Archangel colours and qualities

Ariel: pale pink. *Quality:* Confidence, manifestation. *Crystal:* Rose Quartz

Atrugiel: red, black/smoky. *Quality:* Protection. *Crystal:* Garnet

Azrael: creamy white. *Quality:* Comfort, transition. *Crystal:* Yellow Calcite

Chamuel: pale green. *Quality:* Peace, finder of lost things. *Crystal:* Moldavite Calcite, pale green Fluorite

Gabriel: copper, white. *Quality:* Revelation. *Crystal:* Citrine

Haniel: pale blue, translucent. *Quality:* Harmony, intuition. *Crystal:* Moonstone

Jeremiel: dark purple. *Quality:* Prophecy, inspiration. *Crystal:* Amethyst

Jophiel: dark pink, magenta. *Quality:* Wisdom, beauty. *Crystal:* Rubellite (Pink Tourmaline)

Lucifer: pure white, clear. *Quality:* Transformation. *Crystal:* Anandalite

Melchizedek: silver/gold. *Quality:* Bringing in light. *Crystal:* Angel or Opal Aura Quartz, Rutilated Quartz Metatron: violet, pink, green. *Quality:* Expansion. *Crystal:* Watermelon Tourmaline

Michael: lilac, royal purple, royal blue, gold. *Quality:* Courage. *Crystal:* Lapis Lazuli, Sugilite

Raguel: pale blue, blue-green. *Quality:* Harmonious relationship. *Crystal:* Aquamarine

Raphael: emerald green. *Quality:* Healing. *Crystal:* Emerald, Malachite, Prehnite

Raziel: rainbow colours. *Quality:* Spiritual insight, Akashic keeper. *Crystal:* Clear/Iris Quartz, Rainbow Mayanite

Sandalphon: turquoise. *Quality:* Truth. *Crystal:* Turquoise

Uriel: yellow, red. *Quality:* Ideas. *Crystal:* Amber

Zadkiel: purple, deep indigo blue. *Quality:* Compassion, forgiveness. *Crystal:* Lapis Lazuli, Lilac Celestite

A-Z Directory

Choose 1–4 crystals from an entry when creating your essence.

– A –

Alta major chakra: see page 107

Anchor above and below: Black Kyanite, Black/brown Flint, Blue Flint, Blue Moonstone, Brandenberg Amethyst, Celestobarite, Fulgarite, Gaia Stone, Geothite, Hackmanite, Hubnerite, Kakortokite, Lemurian Jade, Nebula Stone, Nuummite, Prasiolite, Preseli Bluestone, Rutile/Rutilated Quartz, Shaman Quartz, Smoky Rose Quartz, Specular Hematite, White Flint. *Chakra:* base, earth star, Gaia gateway, soma, crown, stellar gateway

> **cosmic anchor:** Azeztulite, Blue Moonstone, Brandenberg Amethyst, Faden Quartz, Flint, Hematite, Kakortokite, Lemurian Jade, Lemurian Seed, Menalite, Prasiolite, Preseli Bluestone, Rutilated Quartz, Rutile, Smoky Elestial Quartz, Smoky Rose Quartz, Specular Hematite, Starseed Quartz, Stellar Beam Calcite, Stibnite, Trigonic Quartz. *Chakra:* soma, crown, stellar gateway

> **shamanic (Earth) anchor:** Black Tourmaline, Boji Stones, Calcite Fairy Stone, Celestobarite, Flint, Fulgarite, Gaia Stone, Hematite, Kakortokite, Lemurian Jade, Leopardskin Jasper, Menalite, Obsidian, Rainforest Jasper, Serpentine, Smoky Brandenberg, Smoky Elestial Quartz, Smoky Quartz. *Chakra:* dantien, sacral, base, earth star, Gaia gateway

Anchor expanded awareness: Brandenberg, Flint, Orange Sphalerite, Rhodozite, Temple Calcite, Trigonic Quartz with Tugtupite or Z-stone *and see grounding stones page 226. Chakra:* earth star, Gaia gateway

Archangel/angelic crystals: Amethyst Aura Quartz, Amphibole, Anandalite (Aurora Quartz), Angel Aura Quartz, Angelite, Angel's Wing Calcite, Blue Celestite, Larimar, Lilac Celestite, Prehnite, Rutilated Quartz, Selenite, Seraphinite, Vera Cruz Amethyst *and see Archangels list pages 193–194*

Astral projection/journeying: Afghanite, Apophyllite, Lodalite, Nuummite, Preseli Bluestone, Scolecite, Sedona Stone, Stibnite, Titanite (Sphene). *Chakra:* third eye, soma, crown, *and see Journeying crystals page 198 and travel page 236*

– B –

Balance left-right brain hemispheres: Crystal Cap Amethyst, Cumberlandite, Eudialyte, Lilac Quartz, Rhodozite, Stromatolite, Trigonic Quartz. *Chakra:* soma

Blockages to spiritual expansion, remove: Amazez, Anandalite, Malachite, Obsidian, Rhodochrosite, Rhomboid Selenite, Selenite

Brain stem: Blue Moonstone, Cradle of Life, Chrysotile, Chrysotile in Serpentine, Eye of the Storm, Kambaba Jasper, Schalenblende, Stromatolite

Brainwaves: Brandenberg Amethyst, Crystal Cap Amethyst, Epidote, Nuummite, Prehnite with Epidote, Pyrite and Sphalerite, Schalenblende, Trigonic Quartz,

Vera Cruz Amethyst, White Heulandite. *Chakra:* third
eye, soma, crown, alta major
Brainwaves, beta: Blue Euclase, Brandenberg Amethyst,
Crystal Cap Amethyst, Spirit Quartz, Vera Cruz
Amethyst. *Chakra:* third eye, crown
Brainwaves, combined alpha and theta state: Amazez,
Anandalite, Auralite 23
Brainwaves, harmonise: Blue Euclase, Brandenberg
Amethyst, Eudialyte, Spirit Quartz
Brainwaves: theta: Brandenberg Amethyst, Trigonic
Quartz

– C –
Causal vortex chakra: see page 111
Consciousness expanding crystals: Amazez, Amphibole
Quartz, Auralite 23, Azeztulite, Bloodstone, Celtic
Quartz, Chevron Amethyst, Clear Brandenberg
Amethyst, Crystal Cap Amethyst, Danburite, Fire and
Ice, Grape Chalcedony, Herkimer Diamond, Hiddenite,
Himalayan Quartz, Lapis Lace, Lilac Quartz, Lodalite,
Lumi Quartz, Mystic Merlinite, Nirvana Quartz, Sacred
Scribe, Satyaloka and Satyamani Quartz, Selenite,
Tanzanite, Temple Calcite, Trigonic Quartz, Vera Cruz
Amethyst
Cosmic wisdom, access: Anandalite, Lemurian Seed,
Nuummite, Petalite, Trigonic

– F –
Fear of expansion, overcome: Amethyst, Auralite 23,

Kammerite, Moqui Marbles (make essence by indirect method), Sunstone-and-Iolite

– G –

Gaia/Mother Earth wisdom: Blue Kyanite, Flint, Gaia's Blood Flint, Herkimer Diamond, Kambaba Jasper, Smoky Quartz

– I –

Intuition openers: Apophyllite, Auralite 23, Boulder Opal, Bytownite (Yellow Labradorite), Golden Herkimer, Labradorite, Lapis Lazuli, Rhomboid Selenite, Tanzine Aura Quartz, White Calcite

– J –

Journeying crystals: Andean Opal, Aztee, Polychrome Jasper, Preseli Bluestone, Scolecite, Sedona Stone, Serpentine, Serpentine in Obsidian, Shaman Quartz, Stibnite, Titanite (Sphene)

– M –

Meditation: Amazez, Amethyst, Ammolite, Ammonite, Anandalite™, Apophyllite, Auralite 23, Azeztulite, Azurite, Bytownite, Celtic Healer, Chevron Amethyst, Elestial Rose Quartz, Herkimer Diamond, Lapis Lazuli, Lemurian Seed, Nirvana Quartz, Petalite, Phenacite, Quartz, Sacred Scribe, Selenite, Smoky Elestial Quartz, Tibetan Quartz, Vera Cruz Amethyst

Multidimensional consciousness: Amazez, Aquitaine

Calcite, Astrophyllite, Auralite 23, Azurite, Cathedral Quartz, Fire and Ice, Grape Chalcedony, Herderite, Indicolite Quartz, Labradorite, Lapis Lazuli, Lemurian Seed, Libyan Gold Tektite, Lodalite, Lumi, Moldavite, Mystic Merlinite, Prairie Tanzanite, Satyamani and Satyaloka Quartz, Shiva Shell, Spectrolite, Starbrary Quartz, Sunset Sodalite, Trigonic Quartz *and see Consciousness expanding above*

Multidimensional travel: Afghanite, Anandalite™, Auralite 23, Aztee, Banded Agate, Blue Moonstone, Brandenberg Amethyst, Celestobarite, Celtic Quartz, Golden Selenite, Kinoite, Novaculite, Nunderite, Orange Creedite, Owyhee Blue Opal, Phantom Quartz, Polychrome Jasper, Preseli Bluestone, Rainbow Moonstone, Sedona Stone, Shaman Quartz, Spectrolite, Spirit Quartz, Tanzanite, Thunder Egg, Titanite (Sphene), Trigonic Quartz, Ussingite, Vivianite, Youngite

– P –

Prohibitions on using psychic sight, release: Apophyllite pyramid, Aquamarine, Astrophyllite, Azurite, Bytownite, Lapis Lazuli, Rhomboid Selenite. *Chakra:* third eye

Protection when travelling: Amazonite, Black Tourmaline, Labradorite, Petrified Wood, Prairie Tanzanite, Shungite. *Disperse around aura.*

Psychic shield: Actinolite, Amphibole, Azotic Topaz, Aztee, Black Tourmaline, Bornite, Bowenite (New Jade), Brandenberg Amethyst, Brazilianite, Celestobarite,

Chlorite Shaman Quartz, Crackled Fire Agate, Fiskenaesset Ruby, Frondellite with Strengite, Gabbro, Graphic Smoky Quartz (Zebra Stone), Hanksite, Iridescent Pyrite, Keyiapo, Labradorite, Lorenzite (Ramsayite), Marcasite, Master Shamanite, Mohave Turquoise, Mohawkite, Owyhee Blue Opal, Polychrome Jasper, Purpurite, Pyromorphite, Quantum Quattro, Red Amethyst, Silver Leaf Jasper, Smoky Amethyst, Smoky Elestial Quartz, Tantalite, Thunder Egg, Valentinite and Stibnite, Xenotine. *Chakra:* third eye. *Disperse around aura.*
'Psychic sponge': Green Aventurine, Healer's Gold, Labradorite, Mohawkite, Shungite, Tantalite. *Chakra:* solar plexus, spleen, third eye. *Or, disperse around aura.*

– S –

Safe space: Apache Tear, Black Tourmaline, Flint, Selenite, Shungite and Clear Quartz, Smoky Quartz
Shamanic journey: Brandenberg Amethyst, Celestobarite, Chrysotile in Serpentine, Graphic Smoky Quartz (Zebra Stone), Leopardskin Jasper, Lodalite, Mount Shasta Opal, Nunderite, Owyhee Blue Opal, Polychrome Jasper, Preseli Bluestone, Scolecite, Serpentine in Obsidian, Shaman Quartz, Smoky Quartz with Aegerine, Stibnite, Titanite (Sphene). *See also Journeying crystals page 198.*
Shamanic realms: Lodalite, Merlinite, Serpentine
Shape shifting: Leopardskin Jasper, Mount Shasta Opal, Serpentine in Obsidian. *Chakra:* soma, third eye
Shield yourself: Black Tourmaline, Healer's Gold,

Mohawkite, Nuummite, Polychrome Jasper, Pyrite, Shieldite, Shungite, Smoky Quartz, Tantalite. *Chakra:* higher heart

Soul star chakra: see page 122

Spiritual guidance: Amethyst, Anandalite, Astrophyllite, Azeztulite, Azurite, Dumortierite, Indicolite Quartz, Kyanite, Lapis Lazuli, Mentor formation, Moldavite, Orange Calcite, Petalite, Phenacite, Pink Phantom Quartz, Smoky Amethyst, Smoky Elestial, Spirit Quartz, Super 7, Tanzanite, Tanzine Aura Quartz, Vivianite

Spiritual success: Ammolite, Anandalite, Boulder Opal, Lapis Lazuli, Moonstone, Morganite, Peridot, Turquoise. *Chakra:* crown chakra

Stellar gateway chakra: *see page 124*

Sudden energy drain: Agate, Apache Tear, Black Tourmaline, Carnelian, Green Aventurine, Green Fluorite, Jade, Labradorite, Polychrome Jasper, Red Jasper, Shungite, Triplite

– V –

Vibrational change, facilitate: Anandalite, Bismuth, Gabbro, Hubnerite, Lemurian Gold Opal, Lemurian Jade, Lemurian Seed, Luxullianite, Montebrasite, Mtrolite, Nunderite, Rainbow Mayanite, Rosophia, Sanda Rosa Azeztulite, Snakeskin Pyrite, Sonora Sunrise, Trigonic Quartz. *Chakra:* higher heart, higher crown. *Or spritz essence around head or environment.*

Emotional and mental healing essences

Changing our response (thinking) to negative events changes our belief (a belief being no more than a thought that one continues to think) and can promote healing because the belief is no longer being fed.

– Janet Bleasdale

Select 1–4 appropriate crystals when creating your essence and add a regulating crystal if the emotional or mental imprint is particularly ingrained or your energy field fragile. If more than four crystals dowse as appropriate, consider using concatenation, see page 70.

– A –

Abandonment: Cassiterite, Chalcanthite, Eye of the Storm, Grape Chalcedony, Mangano Calcite, Prairie Tanzanite, Quantum Quattro, Rhodozaz, Tugtupite. *Chakra:* base, heart

Abuse: Apricot Quartz, Azeztulite with Morganite, Eilat Stone, Honey Opal, Lazurine, Lemurian Jade, Pink Crackle Quartz, Proustite, Red Quartz, Septarian, Smoky Amethyst, Smoky Citrine, Xenotine. *Chakra:* base, sacral

Alienation, overcome: Amphibole Quartz, Bustamite with Sugilite, Champagne Aura Quartz, Gaia Stone. *Chakra:* earth star, solar plexus, soma

Anger, ameliorate: Cinnabar in Jasper, Ethiopian Opal,

Nzuri Moyo. *Chakra:* base, dantien

Anxiety: Eye of the Storm, Galaxyite, Khutnohorite, Lemurian Aquitane Calcite, Lemurian Gold Opal, Nzuri Moyo, Oceanite, Owyhee Blue Opal, Pyrite in Magnesite, Riebekite with Sugilite and Bustamite, Scolecite, Strawberry Quartz, Tanzanite, Thunder Egg, Tremolite, Tugtupite. *Chakra:* earth star, base

– B –

Baggage, releasing emotional: Ajoite, Chrysotile in Serpentine, Cumberlandite, Eclipse Stone, Garnet in Quartz, Golden Healer Quartz, Graphic Smoky Quartz (Zebra Stone), Mount Shasta Opal, Rose Elestial Quartz, Tangerose, Tanzine Aura Quartz, Tremolite, Tugtupite, Wind Fossil Agate, Xenotine. *Chakra:* solar plexus, heart

Beliefs that no longer serve, release: Ancestralite, Cradle of Life (Humankind), Freedom Stone, Geothite, Lakelandite. *Chakra:* past life, third eye

Belonging: Polychrome Jasper. *Chakra:* earth star, base, dantien

Betrayal: Quantum Quattro, Smoky Rose Quartz, Tugtupite

Bigotry, overcome effects of: Tugtupite. *Chakra:* heart

Bitterness: Gaspeite, Hubnerite, Rose Quartz. *Chakra:* heart

Blocked feelings: Indicolite Quartz, Pyrite-and-Sphalerite, Pyrite in Quartz, Rhodonite, Rose Quartz, Tanzine Aura Quartz

Broken heart: Cobalto Calcite, Mangano Vesuvianite,

Rhodochrosite, Tugtupite. *Chakra:* past life, heart
Burnout: Crackled Fire Agate, Marcasite, Poppy Jasper, Quantum Quattro, Que Sera, Strawberry Lemurian. *Chakra:* base, dantien

– C –

Calming emotions: Mount Shasta Opal, Oceanite, Tugtupite
Calming fear: Arsenopyrite, Eilat Stone, Graphic Smoky Quartz (Zebra Stone), Guardian Stone, Khutnohorite, Oceanite, Scolecite, Tangerose, Thunder Egg
Childhood, difficult: Cassiterite, Fenster Quartz, Red Phantom Quartz, Shiva Lingam, Tugtupite, Tugtupite with Nuummite, Voegesite, Youngite. *Chakra:* heart, solar plexus
Clarity, promote: Adamite, Ammolite, Blue Moonstone, Blue Quartz, Chinese Chromium Quartz, Chinese Red Quartz, Datolite, Dumortierite, Green Ridge Quartz, Holly Agate, Judy's Jasper, Lemurian Seed, Leopardskin Jasper, Limonite, Marcasite, Morion, Pearl Spa Dolomite, Purpurite, Rainforest Jasper, Realgar and Orpiment, Scapolite, Seriphos Quartz, Silver Leaf Jasper, Smoky Candle Quartz, Super 7, Tangerine Sun Aura Quartz, Tugtupite. *Chakra:* third eye, alta major, crown
Control freak: Chrysotile, Ice Quartz, Lazulite, Lemurian Aquitane Calcite, Spiders Web Obsidian. *Chakra:* dantien

– D –

Dark moods, ameliorate: Tantalite, Vera Cruz Amethyst.

Chakra: solar plexus, third eye

Defensive walls, dismantle: Calcite Fairy Stone, Eye of the Storm

Detoxify emotions: Golden Danburite, Golden Healer, Rhodolite Garnet, Rhodonite, Seraphinite, Spirit Quartz. *Chakra:* solar plexus

Distress: Eye of the Storm, Lemurian Gold Opal, Owyhee Blue Opal, Tugtupite. *Chakra:* heart

Dysfunctional patterns, dissolve: Alunite, Arfvedsonite, Celadonite, Dumortierite, Fenster Quartz, Garnet in Quartz, Glendonite, Rainbow Covellite, Scheelite, Spiders Web Obsidian, Stellar Beam Calcite

– E –

Egotism: Bixbite, Hematoid Calcite, Lepidocrocite, Rathbunite™, Red Amethyst. *Chakra:* base, dantien

Emotional abuse: Azeztulite with Morganite, Cobalto Calcite, Eilat Stone, Lazurine, Pink Crackle Quartz, Proustite, Tugtupite. *Chakra:* sacral, heart

Emotional alienation: Cassiterite

Emotional angst: Hemimorphite, Rhodonite

Emotional attachment: Brandenberg, Drusy Golden Healer, Hemimorphite, Pink Crackle Quartz, Rainbow Mayanite, Tinguaite

Emotional autonomy: Faden Quartz. *Chakra:* dantien

Emotional balance: Amblygonite, Dalmatian Stone, Eilat Stone

Emotional black hole: Ajoite, Cobalto Calcite, Quantum Quattro. *Chakra:* higher heart

Emotional blackmail: Tugtupite. *Chakra:* solar plexus

Emotional blockages: Aegirine, Botswana Agate, Bowenite (New Jade), Clinohumite, Cobalto Calcite, Eilat Stone, Green Ridge Quartz, Prehnite with Epidote, Pyrite and Sphalerite, Quantum Quattro, Rainbow Mayanite, Rhodozite, Tangerose, Tanzine Aura Quartz. *Chakra:* solar plexus

Emotional blockages from past lives: Aegirine, Datolite, Dumortierite, Graphic Smoky Quartz (Zebra Stone), Prehnite with Epidote, Pyrite and Sphalerite, Quantum Quattro, Rhodozite, Rose Elestial Quartz, Serpentine in Obsidian, *and see Healing page 257. Chakra:* past life, causal vortex

Emotional bondage: Ajoite. *Chakra:* solar plexus

Emotional burnout: Cobalto Calcite, Golden Healer Quartz, Lilac Quartz. *Chakra:* heart

Emotional conditioning: Clevelandite, Drusy Golden Healer, Golden Healer Quartz. *Chakra:* solar plexus, third eye

Emotional debris: Ajoite, Pink Lemurian Seed, Rainbow Mayanite. *Chakra:* solar plexus

Emotional dependency: Cobalto Calcite. *Chakra:* base

Emotional dysfunction: Chinese Red Phantom Quartz, Fenster Quartz, Orange Kyanite. *Chakra:* higher heart

Emotional/emotions: *Chakra:* solar plexus, heart

Emotional equilibrium: Adamite, Merlinite, Quantum Quattro, Rutile with Hematite, Shungite

Emotional exhaustion: Cinnabar in Jasper, Lilac Quartz, Orange River Quartz, Prehnite with Epidote

Emotional healing: Garnet in Quartz, Mount Shasta Opal, Tugtupite, Xenotine

Emotional hooks, remove: Amblygonite, Drusy Golden Healer, Geothite, Golden Danburite, Klinoptilolith, Novaculite, Nunderite, Nuummite, Orange Kyanite, Pyromorphite, Rainbow Mayanite, Tantalite, Tugtupite. *Chakra:* solar plexus

Emotional manipulation: Pink Lemurian Seed, Tantalite. *Chakra:* sacral, solar plexus, third eye

Emotional maturation: Alexandrite, Cobalto Calcite

Emotional negative, destructive attachments: Ajoite, Drusy Golden Healer, Ilmenite, Pink Lemurian Seed, Rainbow Mayanite, Tantalite, Tinguaite. *Chakra:* base, solar plexus

Emotional pain after separation: Aegirine, Eilat Stone, Tugtupite. *Chakra:* higher heart

Emotional patterns: Arfvedsonite, Brandenberg Amethyst, Celadonite, Fenster Quartz, Rainbow Covellite, Scheelite. *Chakra:* solar plexus, base

Emotional recovery: Empowerite, Eye of the Storm, Lilac Quartz. *Chakra:* higher heart

Emotional release: Axinite, Cobalto Calcite, Scheelite. *Chakra:* solar plexus, base, sacral

Emotional, reveal underlying causes of distress: Eye of the Storm, Gaia Stone, Lemurian Gold Opal, Obsidian, Rainbow Obsidian, Richterite, Riebekite with Sugilite and Bustamite, Smoky Amethyst, Snowflake Obsidian. *Chakra:* solar plexus, past life

Emotional security: Mangano Vesuvianite, Oceanite,

Tugtupite. *Chakra:* base, dantien, solar plexus

Emotional shock: Tantalite, Tugtupite. *Chakra:* heart

Emotional shutdown, release: Ice Quartz

Emotional strength: Brazilianite, Mohawkite, Picrolite, Tree Agate. *Chakra:* heart

Emotional stress, dissolve: Cobalto Calcite, Eye of the Storm, Icicle Calcite, Shungite, Tugtupite. *Chakra:* solar plexus

Emotional tension: Strawberry Quartz. *Chakra:* solar plexus

Emotional toxicity: Ajoite, Arsenopyrite, Banded Agate, Champagne Aura Quartz, Drusy Danburite with Chlorite, Valentinite and Stibnite

Emotional trauma: Ajoite, Blue Euclase, Cobalto Calcite, Empowerite, Epidote, Eye of the Storm, Gaia Stone, Grape Chalcedony, Graphic Smoky Quartz (Zebra Stone), Holly Agate, Mangano Vesuvianite, Orange River Quartz, Prairie Tanzanite, Richterite, Tantalite, Tugtupite, Victorite. *Chakra:* solar plexus

Emotional turmoil: Cobalto Calcite, Desert Rose. *Chakra:* base

Emotional wounds, heal: Ajoite, Bustamite, Cassiterite, Cobalto Calcite, Eilat Stone, Gaia Stone, Macedonian Opal, Mookaite Jasper, Orange River Quartz, Piemontite, Rathbunite™, Rhodonite, Rose Quartz, Xenotine. *Chakra:* higher heart

Emotions, frozen feelings: Clevelandite, Diopside, Eilat Stone, Ice Quartz, Scolecite. *Chakra:* solar plexus, heart, heart seed, higher heart

Emotions, restore trust: Clevelandite, Faden Quartz, Xenotine

Emotions, revitalise: Orange River Quartz, Vivianite

Empty nest syndrome: Menalite, Moonstone. *Chakra:* sacral

– F –

Frustration, overcome: Chinese Red Quartz, Poppy Jasper, Pyrite in Magnesite, Rooster Tail Quartz. *Chakra:* base, dantien

– G –

Grief: Aegirine, Ajo Quartz, Blue Drusy Quartz, Cobalto Calcite, Datolite, Diopside, Empowerite, Epidote, Girasol, Indicolite Quartz, Khutnohorite, Mangano Vesuvianite, Quantum Quattro, Ruby in Fuchsite or Kyanite. *Chakra:* higher heart

– H –

Heart trauma: Azeztulite with Morganite, Blue Euclase, Cobalto Calcite, Gaia Stone, Golden Healer, Mangano Vesuvianite, Oceanite, Peanut Wood, Quantum Quattro, Rhodolite Garnet, Rhodonite, Rose Elestial Quartz, Roselite, Ruby Lavender Quartz, Tantalite, Victorite

Heart, unblock: Gaspeite, Golden Healer, Mangano Calcite, Pink Lemurian Seed, Prasiolite, Rhodochrosite, Rhodolite Garnet, Rhodonite, Smoky Rose Quartz, Tugtupite

Helplessness: Actinolite Quartz, Adamite, Brazilianite,

Bronzite, Carnelian, Clevelandite, Covellite, Dumortierite, Kakortokite, Mystic Topaz, Ocean Jasper, Paraiba Tourmaline, Pumice, Quantum Quattro, Tree Agate. *Chakra:* earth star, base, sacral, dantien

– I –

Incest, overcome effects: Cobalto Calcite, Eilat Stone, Golden Healer, Rhodolite Garnet, Tugtupite. *Chakra:* base, sacral, solar plexus.

Inferiority complex: Pyrite in Magnesite, Rhodolite Garnet. *Chakra:* dantien

Inner child: Cobalto Calcite, Dalmatian Stone, Fairy Quartz, Hanksite, Limonite, Pink Crackle Quartz, Quantum Quattro, Spirit Quartz, Voegesite, Youngite. *Chakra:* sacral

Intimacy, lack of: Axinite, Cobalto Calcite, Datolite, Rhodochrosite, Rhodonite, Rose Azeztulite, Rose Quartz, Rosophia, Tugtupite

Intolerance: Pyrite in Magnesite, Rose Quartz

– J –

Jealousy: Eclipse Stone, Heulandite, Rainbow Mayanite, Rosophia, Tugtupite, Zircon. *Chakra:* heart

Judgementalism: Green Heulandite, Mohawkite, Tantalite. *Chakra:* dantien

– L –

Left-right confusion: Black Moonstone, Bustamite with Sugilite, Rainbow Moonstone. *Chakra:* third eye, crown, alta major

Letting go past: Axinite, Fenster Quartz, Fulgarite, Green Diopside, Kakortokite, Kimberlite, Lepidocrocite, Nuummite, Paraiba Tourmaline, Pumice, Scheelite, Zircon. *Chakra:* solar plexus, heart, past life

Limiting patterns of behaviour: Ajoite, Amphibole, Arfvedsonite, Atlantasite, Barite, Botswana Agate, Bronzite, Cassiterite, Celadonite, Chlorite Shaman Quartz, Crackled Fire Agate, Dalmatian Stone, Datolite, Dream Quartz, Dumortierite, Epidote, Garnet in Quartz, Glendonite, Halite, Hanksite, Hematoid Calcite, Honey Phantom Calcite, Indicolite Quartz, Kinoite, Marcasite, Merlinite, Nuummite, Oligocrase, Owyhee Blue Opal, Pearl Spa Dolomite, Porphyrite (Chinese Letter Stone), Quantum Quattro, Rainbow Covellite, Scheelite, Spiders Web Obsidian, Stellar Beam Calcite. *Chakra:* base, sacral, dantien, solar plexus, past life

– M –

Mental abuse: Apricot Quartz, Lazurine, Proustite, Tugtupite with Nuummite, Yellow Crackle Quartz, Xenotine

Mental agitation: Amethyst, Strawberry Quartz, Youngite

Mental attachments: Aegerine, Banded Agate, Blue Halite, Botswana Agate, Lemurian Seed, Limonite, Pyrolusite, Smoky Amethyst, Yellow Phantom Quartz. *Chakra:* third eye

Mental blockages: Auralite 23, Fluorite, Molybdenite,

Rhodozite

Mental breakdown: Molybdenite, Novaculite, Quantum Quattro, Youngite. *Chakra:* third eye, crown

Mental clarity: Holly Agate, Merkabite Calcite, Moldau Quartz, Poldervaarite, Realgar and Orpiment, Sacred Scribe, Star Hollandite, Temple Calcite, Thompsonite

Mental cleansing: Black Kyanite, Blue Quartz, Fluorite, Hungarian Quartz

Mental conditioning, rigid: Drusy Golden Healer, Pholocomite, Rainbow Covellite *and see patterns page 213. Chakra:* third eye, crown

Mental confusion: Aegerine, Blue Halite, Blue Quartz, Hematoid Calcite, Limonite, Pholocomite, Poldervaarite, Richterite

Mental detox: Amechlorite, Banded Agate, Drusy Quartz on Sphalerite, Eye of the Storm, Larvikite, Pyrite in Magnesite, Rainbow Covellite, Richterite, Shungite, Smoky Quartz with Aegerine, Spirit Quartz, Tantalite

Mental dexterity/flexibility, improve: Brucite, Bushman Quartz, Coprolite, Green Ridge Quartz, Kimberlite, Limonite, Molybdenite, Seriphos Quartz, Tiffany Stone, Titanite (Sphene). *Chakra:* third eye, crown

Mental dysfunction: Alunite, Star Hollandite, Titanite (Sphene)

Mental exhaustion: Cinnabar in Jasper, Marcasite, Spectrolite

Mental focus: Sacred Scribe (Russian Lemurian)

Mental implants: Amechlorite, Blue Halite, Brandenberg, Cryolite, Drusy Golden Healer, Holly

Agate, Ilmenite, Lemurian Aquitane Calcite, Novaculite, Nuummite, Pholocomite, Tantalite

Mental sabotage: Agrellite, Amphibole, Lemurian Aquitane Calcite, Mohawkite, Paraiba Tourmaline, Tantalite, Yellow Scapolite

Mental strength: Plancheite

Mental, undue influence, remove: Limonite, Novaculite, Tantalite

Mental upheaval: Guinea Fowl Jasper

Mind, butterfly: Amazez, Auralite 23, Fluorite, Tantalite

Mind chatter, switch off: Auralite 23, Bytownite, Rhodozite, Rhomboid Selenite, Richterite, Scheelite. See Over-thinking, page 214.

Mind control: Cryolite, Drusy Golden Healer, Pholocomite, Thunder Egg

Mind, malicious thoughts, release: Hemimorphite, Pholocomite, Scolecite

Mind, negative thought patterns: Amphibole, Arfvedsonite, Celadonite, Dumortierite, Nuummite, Owyhee Blue Opal, Rainbow Covellite, Scheelite, Scolecite

– N –

Narrow-mindedness: Kundalini Quartz. *Chakra:* base, higher heart

Neurotic patterns: Arfvedsonite, Celadonite, Greenlandite, Porphyrite (Chinese Letter Stone), Rainbow Covellite, Scheelite. *Chakra:* solar plexus

Nurturing, lack of: Amblygonite, Bornite on Silver,

Calcite Fairy Stone, Clevelandite, Cobalto Calcite, Drusy Blue Quartz, Flint, Jade, Jasper, Lazurine, Menalite, Mount Shasta Opal, Ocean Jasper, Prasiolite, Rose Quartz, Ruby Lavender Quartz, Septarian, Super 7, Tree Agate, Tugtupite. *Chakra:* higher heart, base

– O –

Obsessive thoughts: Ammolite, Auralite 23, Barite, Bytownite, Scolecite, Spirit Quartz, Tantalite. *Chakra:* third eye, crown

Outworn patterns: Amphibole, Arfvedsonite, Brandenberg Amethyst, Celadonite, Garnet in Quartz, Owyhee Blue Opal, Porphyrite (Chinese Letter Stone), Quantum Quattro, Rainbow Covellite, Rainbow Mayanite, Scheelite, Stibnite. *Chakra:* earth star, base, sacral, solar plexus, third eye

Over-attachment: Drusy Golden Healer, Rainbow Mayanite, Tantalite, Tinguaite. *Chakra:* solar plexus, navel (tummy button)

Over-thinking: Amazez, Auralite 23, Bytownite, Creedite, Dalmatian Stone, Rhomboid Selenite. *Chakra:* third eye

– P –

Painful feelings, assimilate: Khutnohorite, Tugtupite. *Chakra:* heart

Psychosomatic disease: Andescine Labradorite, Angel's Wing Calcite, Astraline, Azeztulite with Morganite, Azotic Topaz, Benitoite, Dumortierite, Fire Obsidian,

Gaia Stone, Golden Danburite, Icicle Calcite, Larvikite, Ocean Blue Jasper, Roselite, Snakeskin Pyrite, Titanite (Sphene), Voegesite. *Chakra:* third eye, higher heart

– R –

Resentment: Eclipse Stone, Eudialyte, Rose Quartz. *Chakra:* base, dantien

– S –

Sabotage, self: Lemurian Aquitane Calcite, Mohawkite, Scapolite, Scheelite

Scapegoating behaviour: Champagne Aura Quartz, Mohawkite, Scapolite, Smoky Amethyst

Security issues: Chinese Red Quartz, Eye of the Storm, Nzuri Moyo, Prairie Tanzanite. *Chakra:* base

Shadow, integrate: Kammerite, Morion, Proustite, Smoky Lemurian Seed, Voegesite

Speak out: Blue Lace Agate, Honey Opal, Lapis Lace, Titanite (Sphene), Xenotine. *Chakra:* throat

Subconscious blocks: Lepidocrocite, Molybdenite in Quartz, Smoky Elestial Quartz, Smoky Spirit Quartz. *Chakra:* dantien, soul star, stellar gateway, causal vortex, third eye, soma

Suicidal tendencies: Brandenberg Amethyst, Citrine, Pink Petalite, Selenite

– T –

Thought form, disperse: Aegerine, Firework Obsidian, Nuummite, Rainbow Mayanite, Scolecite, Smoky

Amethyst, Smoky Citrine, Spectrolite, Stibnite

Thoughts racing: Auralite 23, Blue Selenite, Pearl Spa Dolomite, Rhomboid Calcite, Scolecite

EMF and Personal Protection

essences

The speculative fears of mobile phones being a danger to health in the long run seem to be coming true. A latest study talks about the harmful effects of not just using mobile phones but also the radiation from mobile phone towers. Radiation from mobile phones and towers poses serious health risks, including loss of memory, lack of concentration, disturbance in the digestive system and sleep disturbances. Study on the hazards posed by mobile phones also reported that the damages may not be lethal for humans, but they are worse for birds and insects as well. The studies have attributed the radiation effects to the disappearance of butterflies, bees, insects and sparrows.
– H.D. Khanna and R.K. Joshi[7]

Electromagnetic fields (EMFs) are present everywhere in the environment, but are invisible to the human eye. The subtle but detectable electromagnetic field given off by power lines, technology and electrical equipment creates electromagnetic smog that may have an adverse effect on sensitive people giving rise to a number of symptoms. Natural electric fields build up through electrical charges associated with thunderstorms and certain geomagnetic anomalies but most detrimental electromagnetic fields are man-made, produced by electrically charged objects. An electromagnetic field is created by differences in voltage; the higher the voltage, the stronger the field and the further its effect radiates.

Effects: In those who are electrosensitive, EMFs may create physiological and psychological problems ranging from energy depletion to severe mood swings, hormone imbalances to metabolic syndrome, chronic fatigue to cancer, short-term memory loss or more serious cognitive dysfunction. The adrenal glands can be stuck in permanent 'fight or flight' mode, the immune system may be disabled and the lymphatic system fails. Many aspects of human metabolism, from the ingestion of nutrients to detoxification and the immune response depend on well-functioning bioelectric processes. The wide-ranging symptoms and effects may be particularly significant for children. (See *Crystal Prescriptions volume 3* for symptoms and research studies.)

Solutions: Rubbing crystal essences on specific chakras helps to strengthen your energy field, which is then better equipped to resist the ill-effects. Essences can also be applied to counteract the detrimental effects. Other solutions to the problems are to drink 1–2 litres of Shungite Water (see page 66) a day, or create a preventative electrosensitive essence to be used daily.

Chakras: Gaia gateway, earth star, base, sacral, dantien, soma, alta major (use access point at base of skull), crown.

Never, ever, take a mobile phone or tablet into your bedroom at night.

Personal Protection

Crystals that protect against EMF emanations will also protect your personal space, and yourself, from detrimental vibes, toxicity and ill-wishing. *See Crystal Prescriptions volume 5: Space clearing, Feng Shui and Psychic Protection* and the A-Z directory.

A-Z Directory

Choose 1–4 crystals from an entry or combined entries when creating your essence.

– A –

Adrenals: see Stress and PTSD

Alzheimer's and mental confusion: Blue Obsidian, Eudialyte, Kunzite, Lepidolite, Purple Tourmaline, Rose Quartz, Rutilated Quartz, Shungite, Sodalite. *Chakra: third eye. Disperse at base of skull.*

Antisocial behaviour/aggression: Amethyst, Blizzard Stone, Bloodstone, Carnelian, Eye of the Storm, Rose Quartz, Ruby, Sardonyx, Selenite, Sodalite. *Disperse in the environment.*

Anti-static: Amber, Fire Agate, Lepidolite, Quartz, Rose Quartz, Shungite, Sodalite, Tourmaline. *Disperse around aura.*

Anxiety: see Stress and PTSD page 286

Atmospheric pollutants, remove: Amber, Black Tourmaline, Chlorite Quartz, Diamond, Elestial Quartz, Fulgarite, Graphite, Halite, Hanksite, Heulandite, Natrolite, Nuummite, Orgonite, Paraiba Tourmaline, Pollucite, Pyrite and Sphalerite, Quantum Quattro, Scolecite, Shaman Quartz, Shieldite, Shungite, Smoky Quartz, Sodalite, Stilbite, Thompsonite, Turquoise. *Chakra: earth star. Or disperse around environment.*

Autoimmune diseases: Aquamarine, Bastnasite, Brandenberg Amethyst, Chinese Red Quartz, Diaspore,

Gabbro, Golden Healer Quartz, Granite, Mookaite Jasper, Paraiba Tourmaline, Quantum Quattro, Que Sera, Rhodonite, Rosophia, Shungite, Tangerose, Titanite (Sphene), Winchite. *Chakra:* dantien, higher heart

Autonomic nervous system: Alexandrite, Amazonite, Amber, Ametrine, Anglesite, Aventurine, Bloodstone, Charoite, Merlinite, Quantum Quattro, Que Sera, Sunstone, Tourmaline. *Chakra:* dantien

– B –

Biological clock disturbances: Fluorapatite, Golden Healer Quartz, Kambaba Jasper, Menalite, Moonstone, Preseli Bluestone, Stromatolite. *Chakra:* dantien, higher heart, third eye or alta major (base of skull)

Biomagnetic field destabilised: Ajoite, Anandalite, Galena (wash hands after use, make essence by indirect method), Kyanite, Lepidolite, Magnetite, Orgonite, Preseli Bluestone, Quartz, Shungite, Sodalite, *and see Aura page 108. Chakra:* dantien, solar plexus

Biomagnetic field, realign/strengthen: Anandalite, Angelinite, Astraline, Celtic Quartz, Ethiopian Opal, Flint, Galena (wash hands after use, make essence by indirect method), Gold in Quartz, Golden Healer Quartz, Magnetite, Poldarvarite, Pollucite, Preseli Bluestone, Quantum Quattro, Que Sera, Shungite, Sodalite

Bone-marrow disorders: Blue John, Cradle of Life, Fluorite, Geothite, Lapis Lazuli, Onyx, Violet-purple Fluorite

Breathing disorders: Blue Aragonite, Blue Crackle Quartz, Hanksite, Morganite, Moss Agate, Riebekite with

Sugilite and Bustamite, Tremolite, Vanadinite. *Chakra:* dantien, heart

– C –

Cancer: Amethyst, Annabergite, Azeztulite, Azurite with Malachite, Bloodstone, Carnelian, Chalcopyrite, Champagne Aura Quartz, Cobaltite, Covellite, Cuprite with Chrysocolla, Diamond, Eilat Stone, Emerald, Fluorapatite, Fluorite, Gabbro, Gold in Quartz, Golden Healer Quartz, Green Ridge Quartz, Hematite, Heulandite, Klinoptilolith, Lapis Lazuli, Lepidolite, Magnetite (Lodestone) with Smoky Quartz, Malachite, Malacolla, Melanite Garnet, Moonstone, Natrolite, Obsidian, Petalite, Pollucite, Quantum Quattro, Que Sera, Red Jasper, Reinerite, Rhodochrosite, Rhodozite, Sapphire, Scolecite, Selenite, Seraphinite, Shungite, Smoky Elestial Quartz, Smoky Quartz, Sodalite, Sonora Sunrise, Spinel, Stilbite, Sugilite, Thompsonite, Tourmaline, Ullmanite, Uvarovite, Xenotine

Cancer, support during treatment: Amethyst Spirit Quartz, Bixbite, Black Diopside, Brandenberg Amethyst, Cassiterite, Cathedral Quartz, Cobolto Calcite, Dendritic Chalcedony, Epidote, Eye of the Storm, Green Ridge Quartz, Hemimorphite, Icicle Calcite, Lemurian Jade, Paraiba Tourmaline, Quantum Quattro, Que Sera, Reinerite, Rhodozite, Sonora Sunrise, Sugilite, Tremolite, Winchite

Candida: Carnelian, Dendritic Chalcedony, Green Calcite, Lepidolite, Moss Agate, Quartz, Snowflake

Obsidian, Zincite. Bathe in the essence.

Cell phones, protection against: Amazonite, Black Tourmaline, Diamond, Orgonite, Rose Quartz, Shieldite, Shungite, Smoky Elestial Quartz, Smoky Quartz, Sodalite. *Disperse around ears.*

Chemical pollution: Amber, Chlorite Quartz, Granite, Halite, Hanksite, Pumice, Quantum Quattro, Shungite, Smoky Elestial Quartz, Smoky Quartz, Tantalite

Clearing 'bad vibes': Amazonite, Amber, Amethyst, Aventurine, Black Tourmaline, Chlorite Quartz, Fluorite, Fulgarite, Graphic Smoky Quartz, Iron Pyrite, Kyanite, Lepidolite, Magnetite, Quartz, Rose Quartz, Selenite, Smoky Elestial Quartz, Smoky Quartz, Selenite, Shieldite, Shungite, Tantalite, Tektite

Close down and ground: Agate, Black Tourmaline, Bloodstone, Boji Stones, Dravide (Brown) Tourmaline, Fire Agate, Galena, Hematite, Magnetite, Obsidian, Smoky Quartz, Sodalite, Tourmalinated Quartz, Unakite. *Chakra:* base or earth star

Computer stress: Amazonite, Amber, Aventurine, Chlorite Quartz, Eye of the Storm, Fluorite, Fulgarite, Galena (*caution: toxic*), Lepidolite, Orgonite, Purple Sugilite, Rose Quartz, Shieldite, Shungite, Smoky Quartz, Sodalite, Sugilite, Tektite. *Chakra:* higher heart

– D –

Dementia: Anthrophyllite, Atlantasite, Holly Agate, Stichtite, Stichtite and Serpentine. *Chakra:* third eye, alta major

Electrical systems of body, rebalance: Amber, Amblygonite, Cavansite, Galena (*caution: toxic*), Golden Healer Quartz, Montebrasite, Orgonite, Pollucite, Shiva Lingam, Shungite

Electromagnetic antidote: Ajoite in Shattuckite, Amazonite, Amber, Auralite 23, Aventurine, Black Moonstone, Black Tourmaline, Black Tourmaline in Quartz, Blizzard Stone, Bloodstone, Chlorite Quartz, Diamond, Flint, Fluorapatite, Fluorite, Fulgarite, Gabbro, Galena (*caution: toxic*), Graphic Smoky Quartz, Herkimer Diamond, Jasper, Klinoptilolith, Lepidolite, Malachite, Native Copper, Natrolite, Obsidian, Orgonite, Phlogopite, Pollucite, Pyrite in Quartz, Quantum Quattro, Quartz, Que Sera, Red Amethyst, Rose Quartz, Scolecite, Shieldite, Shungite, Smoky Quartz, Sodalite, Stilbite, Thunder Egg, Yellow Kunzite

Electromagnetic field, regulate personal: Ajoite in Shattuckite, Amazonite, Amber, Auralite 23, Black Moonstone, Celtic Quartz, Champagne Aura Quartz, Eye of the Storm, Fluorapatite, Fluorite, Fulgarite, Gabbro, Galena (*caution: toxic*), Golden Healer Quartz, Montebrasite, Poppy Jasper, Preseli Bluestone, Quantum Quattro, Que Sera, Rose Quartz, Shungite. *Chakra:* earth star, base. *Or disperse in environment.*

Electromagnetic pollution, protect against: Ajoite in Shattuckite, Amazonite, Amber, Andara Glass, Black Moonstone, Black Tourmaline, Blizzard Stone, Champagne Aura Quartz, Chlorite Quartz, Diamond,

Flint, Fluorite, Gabbro, Galena (*caution: toxic*), Graphic Smoky Quartz, Hackmanite, Herkimer Diamond, Klinoptilolith, Kunzite, Lepidolite, Malachite, Marble, Morion, Native Copper, Orgonite, Phlogopite, Poppy Jasper, Quartz, Que Sera, Red Amethyst, Rose Quartz, Shieldite, Shungite, Smoky Elestial Quartz, Smoky Herkimer Diamond, Smoky Quartz, Sodalite, Tantalite, Thunder Egg. *Chakra:* earth star, base. *Or disperse in environment or around house.*

– F –

Free radicals, damage from: Aquamarine, Brochantite, Diaspore (Zultanite), Klinoptilolith, Selenite, Shungite. *Chakra:* higher heart

Free radicals, remove: Aquamarine, Diaspore, Klinoptilolith, Shungite, Super Seven

– G –

Geopathic stress: Amazonite, Amethyst, Black Tourmaline, Brown Jasper, Champagne Aura Quartz, Chlorite Quartz, Eye of the Storm, Flint, Gabbro, Granite, Graphic Smoky Quartz, Ironstone, Kunzite, Labradorite, Marble, Orgonite, Preseli Bluestone, Pyrite and Sphalerite, Quartz, Riebekite with Sugilite and Bustamite, Selenite, Shieldite, Shungite, Smoky Amethyst, Smoky Elestial, Smoky Quartz, Sodalite, Tantalite, Tektite, Thunder Egg, Trummer Jasper. *Chakra:* earth star. *Or disperse around corners of house.*

Giddiness: Boji Stones, Emerald, Hematite, Pearl,

Quartz, Sodalite. *Chakra:* dantien

Grounding: Ajo Quartz, Amphibole, Aztee, Banded Agate, Basalt, Blue Aragonite, Boji Stones, Bronzite, Brown Jasper, Bustamite, Calcite Fairy Stone, Champagne Aura Quartz, Chlorite Quartz, Cloudy Quartz, Dalmatian Stone, Empowerite, Fire Agate, Flint, Gabbro, Granite, Healer's Gold, Hematite, Hematoid Calcite, Herkimer Diamond, Honey Phantom Quartz, Kambaba Jasper, Keyiapo, Lazulite, Lemurian Jade, Lemurian Seed, Leopardskin Serpentine, Libyan Gold Tektite, Limonite, Luxullianite, Marcasite, Merlinite, Mohawkite, Novaculite, Nunderite, Peanut Wood, Pearl Spa Dolomite, Petrified Wood, Poppy Jasper, Preseli Bluestone, Purpurite, Pyrite in Magnesite, Quantum Quattro, Red Jasper, Rutile with Hematite, Schalenblende, Serpentine in Obsidian, Smoky Elestial Quartz, Smoky Herkimer, Smoky Quartz, Sodalite, Steatite, Stromatolite. *Chakra:* base, earth star, dantien

Group, containing your energies when in one: Black Tourmaline, Brown (Dravide) Tourmaline, Healer's Gold, Labradorite, Prehnite

– H –

High frequency communication aerials, microwaves, infrared and radar: Amazonite, Amethyst, Black Moonstone, Black Tourmaline, Chlorite Quartz, Fluorite, Gabbro, Germanium, Granite, Graphic Smoky Quartz, Hematite, Herkimer Diamond, Klinoptilolith, Malachite, Orgonite, Reinerite, Shieldite, Shungite, Smoky Elestial

Quartz, Smoky Quartz, Sodalite, Sphalerite, Tourmalinated Quartz, Tourmaline, Yellow Kunzite, Zeolite. *Disperse around site or between you and the site.*

– I –

Ill-wishing, protection against: Actinolite, Amethyst, Black Tourmaline, Blue Chalcedony, Bronzite (use with caution as may amplify), Crackled Fire Agate, Fire Agate, Galena (*caution: potentially toxic*), Limonite, Master Shamanite, Mohawkite, Nunderite, Nuummite, Purpurite, Richterite, Rose Quartz, Tantalite, Tugtupite. *Chakra:* throat

Ill-wishing, return to source so that effect is understood: Beryl, Bronzite, Calcite, Chalcedony, Quartz, Selenite, Silver

Insomnia/disturbed sleep patterns: Ajoite, Ajoite with Shattuckite, Amethyst, Bloodstone, Candle Quartz, Celestite, Charoite, Glendonite, Hematite, Howlite, Khutnohorite, Lapis Lazuli, Lepidolite, Magnetite (Lodestone) [*Disperse at head and foot of bed*], Moonstone, Mount Shasta Opal, Muscovite, Ocean Jasper, Owyhee Blue Opal, Petrified Wood, Pink Sunstone, Poldarvarite, Rosophia, Selenite, Shungite, Sodalite, Tektite, Topaz, Zoisite. *Drop on to pillow or disperse around head.*

Insomnia from geopathic/electromagnetic stress/pollution: Black Tourmaline, Chlorite Quartz, Crystal Cap Amethyst, Eye of the Storm, Gabbro, Guinea Fowl Jasper, Herkimer Diamond, Klinoptilolith, Labradorite, Marble, Ocean Jasper, Orgonite, Red Amethyst, Shieldite,

Shungite, Smoky Herkimer Diamond, Smoky Quartz, Sodalite, Spectrolite, Tektite, Thunder Egg. *Disperse round bed and/or drop around the four corners of the room or house, depending on how strong the stress.*

Insomnia from overactive mind: Amethyst, Auralite 23, Blue Selenite, Bytownite (Yellow Labradorite), Crystal Cap Amethyst, Rhodozite, Sodalite, Spectrolite. *Chakra:* third eye

Insomnia from stress: Amethyst, Chrysoprase, Eye of the Storm, Lemurian Gold Opal, Riebekite with Sugilite and Bustamite, Rose Quartz, Shungite, Sodalite, Tektite *and see Stress and PTSD page 286. Chakra:* higher heart

– M –

Microwaves: Amazonite, Amethyst, Black Moonstone, Black Tourmaline, Chlorite Quartz, Fluorite, Gabbro, Germanium, Granite, Graphic Smoky Quartz, Hematite, Herkimer Diamond, Klinoptilolith, Malachite, Orgonite, Reinerite, Shieldite, Shungite, Smoky Elestial Quartz, Smoky Quartz, Sodalite, Sphalerite, Tourmalinated Quartz, Tourmaline, Yellow Kunzite, Zeolite. *Disperse around site or between you and the site.*

– P –

Panic attacks: See Addictions page 186

Primary essence to combat electrosensitivity: Black Tourmaline, Green Aventurine, Rose Quartz, Selenite, Shungite, Smoky Quartz. *Disperse around the aura on waking and before sleeping.*

Environmental and Earth-healing essences

Layouts do not have to be large to be effective. Small crystals can be laid into protective and cleansing layouts such as the triangle, pentacle or the zigzag, or into energizing layouts such as the spiral or sunburst. As some high vibration crystals can be expensive, placing one of these in the centre and adding clear Quartz points facing away from the centre amplifies and channels the energy outwards.

Judy Hall, *Earth Blessings*

Rather than laying expensive or difficult to source crystals in a grid, you can drip essences into a grid pattern or on to one larger crystal to protect and heal your environment. Using Flint, Smoky or Clear Quartz helps to anchor the energetic grid.[8]

Choose 1–4 crystals from an entry when creating your essence.

A-Z Directory

– C –

Chemical pollution: Chlorite Quartz, Quantum Quattro, Shungite, Smoky Elestial Quartz, Tantalite. *Disperse around site and into earth.*

Clearing 'bad vibes': Amazonite, Amber, Amethyst, Aventurine, Black Tourmaline, Chlorite Quartz, Fluorite, Fulgarite, Graphic Smoky Quartz, Iron Pyrite, Kyanite, Lepidolite, Magnetite, Quartz, Selenite, Shieldite, Shungite, Smoky Elestial Quartz, Smoky Quartz, Tantalite, Tektite. *Disperse around site and into earth.*

Computer stress: Amazonite, Amber, Aventurine, Chlorite Quartz, Eye of the Storm, Fluorite, Fulgarite, Galena *(caution: toxic)*, Lepidolite, Orgonite, Purple Sugilite, Rose Quartz, Shieldite, Shungite, Smoky Quartz, Sodalite, Sugilite, Tektite. *Chakra:* higher heart. *Disperse around aura.*

– D –

Detoxification: Amber, Amechlorite, Amethyst, Anhydrite, Apache Tear, Aventurine, Azurite, Banded Agate, Barite, Bastnasite, Bloodstone, Chalk, Chlorite, Chlorite Quartz, Chrysoprase, Conichalcite, Coprolite, Covellite, Cuprite with Chrysocolla, Dendritic Agate, Diaspore, Emerald, Eye of the Storm, Fire Obsidian, Galena *(caution: toxic)*, Golden Danburite, Golden Healer Quartz, Graphic Smoky Quartz, Green Garnet, Greensand, Halite, Hanksite, Herkimer Diamond,

Hypersthene, Iolite, Jade, Jamesonite, Jet, Kambaba Jasper, Larvikite, Malachite, Merlinite, Mica, Obsidian, Ocean Jasper, Orgonite, Phlogopite, Poppy Jasper, Pumice, Quantum Quattro, Que Sera, Rainbow Covellite, Richterite, Ruby, Seraphinite, Shungite, Smoky Elestial Quartz, Smoky Quartz, Smoky Quartz with Aegerine, Stilbite, Sulphur, Sulphur in Quartz, Thunder Egg, Tiger Eye, Topaz, Tree Agate, Turquoise, Zoisite. *Chakra:* solar plexus, earth star, base. *Disperse around site and into earth.*

– E –

Earth-healers: Anandalite, Ancestralite, Aragonite, Black Tourmaline, Brandenberg, Bumble Bee Jasper, Celtic Quartz, Citrine, Clear Quartz, Eye of the Storm (Judy's Jasper), Fire and Ice, Flint, Golden Healer Quartz, Granite, Graphic Smoky Quartz, Halite, Hanksite, Herkimer Diamond, Malachite, Menalite, Preseli Bluestone, Purpurite, Rhodochrosite, Rhodozite, Rose Quartz, Selenite, Shiva Lingam, Smoky Elestial Quartz, Smoky Quartz, Spirit Quartz, Tangerine Dream Lemurians, Trigonic Quartz. *Disperse around site and into earth.*

Electromagnetic: see EMF and Geopathic stress page 225
EMF antidotes: Ajoite in Shattuckite, Amazonite, Amber, Auralite 23, Aventurine, Black Moonstone, Black Tourmaline, Black Tourmaline in Quartz, Blizzard Stone, Bloodstone, Celtic Golden Healer, Chlorite Quartz, Diamond, Flint, Fluorapatite, Fluorite, Fulgarite, Gabbro, Galena (*caution: toxic*), Graphic Smoky Quartz, Herkimer

Diamond, Jasper, Klinoptilolith, Lepidolite, Malachite, Native Copper, Natrolite, Obsidian, Orgonite, Phlogopite, Pollucite, Pyrite in Quartz, Quantum Quattro, Quartz, Que Sera, Red Amethyst, Rose Quartz, Scolecite, Shieldite, Shungite, Smoky Quartz, Sodalite, Stilbite, Thompsonite, Thunder Egg, Yellow Kunzite

Electromagnetic field, regulate personal: Ajoite in Shattuckite, Amazonite, Amber, Auralite 23, Black Moonstone, Celtic Golden Healer, Champagne Aura Quartz, Eye of the Storm, Fluorapatite, Fluorite, Fulgarite, Gabbro, Galena (*caution: toxic*), Golden Healer Quartz, Montebrasite, Poppy Jasper, Preseli Bluestone, Quantum Quattro, Que Sera, Rose Quartz, Shungite. *Chakra*: earth star, base. *Or disperse around aura or in environment.*

EMF antidotes: Ajoite in Shattuckite, Amazonite, Amber, Auralite 23, Aventurine, Black Moonstone, Black Tourmaline, Black Tourmaline in Quartz, Blizzard Stone, Bloodstone, Celtic Golden Healer, Chlorite Quartz, Diamond, Flint, Fluorapatite, Fluorite, Fulgarite, Gabbro, Galena (*caution: toxic*), Graphic Smoky Quartz, Herkimer Diamond, Jasper, Klinoptilolith, Lepidolite, Malachite, Native Copper, Natrolite, Obsidian, Orgonite, Phlogopite, Pollucite, Pyrite in Quartz, Quantum Quattro, Quartz, Que Sera, Red Amethyst, Rose Quartz, Scolecite, Shieldite, Shungite, Smoky Quartz, Sodalite, Stilbite, Thompsonite, Thunder Egg, Yellow Kunzite

Environment, improve: Amazonite, Aragonite, Black Tourmaline, Chlorite Quartz, Eye of the Storm, Golden

Healer Quartz, Malachite, Orgonite, Poppy Jasper, Quartz, Rose Quartz, Selenite, Smoky Quartz, White or Rose Elestial Quartz. *Disperse around site and into earth.*

Environmental diseases: Chlorite Quartz, Drusy Quartz on Sphalerite, Eye of the Storm, Feldspar, Golden Healer Quartz, Marble, Orgonite, Petrified Wood, Poppy Jasper, Preseli Bluestone, Quartz, Shieldite, Shungite, Smoky Elestial Quartz, *and see Geopathic stress page 225. Chakra:* earth star, higher heart. *Or disperse in environment.*

Environmental harmony, create: Grape Chalcedony, Khutnohorite, Rose Quartz, Sardonyx, Selenite

Environmental pollution: Alunite, Amber, Anhydrite, Black Tourmaline, Champagne Aura Quartz, Chlorite Quartz, Eye of the Storm, Flint, Golden Healer Quartz, Graphic Smoky Quartz, Halite, Hanksite, Labradorite, Moss Agate, Orgonite, Phlogopite, Poppy Jasper, Que Sera, Selenite, Shieldite, Shungite, Smoky Elestial Quartz, Smoky Quartz, Sulphur, Sulphur in Quartz, Tantalite, Thunder Egg, Trummer Jasper, Zincite. *Chakra:* earth star. *Disperse in earth or around house.*

– G –

Geopathic stress: Amazonite, Amethyst, Black Tourmaline, Brown Jasper, Champagne Aura Quartz, Chlorite Quartz, Eye of the Storm, Flint, Gabbro, Granite, Graphic Smoky Quartz, Ironstone, Kunzite, Labradorite, Marble, Orgonite, Preseli Bluestone, Pyrite and Sphalerite, Quartz, Riebekite with Sugilite and Bustamite, Selenite, Shieldite, Shungite, Smoky

Amethyst, Smoky Elestial, Smoky Quartz, Sodalite, Tantalite, Tektite, Thunder Egg, Trummer Jasper. *Chakra:* earth star. *Or disperse around corners of house.*

– H –

Headache from negative environmental factors/electromagnetic stress: Galena (*caution: toxic*), Smoky Quartz, Tektite

Home harmonising stones:

Create essence at new moon:

To bring more love into the home: Cobalto Calcite, Danburite, Larimar, Mangano Calcite, Pink Tourmaline, Rhodochrosite, Rose Quartz, Selenite

To clear negativity: Black Tourmaline, Shungite, Smoky Quartz

To create peace and harmony: Eye of the Storm, Larimar, Porcelain Jasper, Selenite

To create well-being and prosperity: Aventurine, Citrine

To encourage everyone to get along with each other: Citrine, Eye of the Storm, Moss Agate *Create essence at full moon:*

– I –

Insomnia from negative environmental influences: Black Tourmaline, Bloodstone, Champagne Aura Quartz, Klinoptilolith, Lepidolite, Marble, Orgonite, Shungite, Smoky Elestial Quartz, Smoky Quartz, Tantalite, Trummer Jasper, Turquoise. *Disperse essence around the*

four corners of the room.
Irritant filter: Limestone, Pumice, Rhodochrosite. *Chakra:* dantien

– M –

Microwaves: Amazonite, Amethyst, Black Moonstone, Black Tourmaline, Chlorite Quartz, Fluorite, Gabbro, Germanium, Granite, Graphic Smoky Quartz, Hematite, Herkimer Diamond, Klinoptilolith, Malachite, Orgonite, Reinerite, Shieldite, Shungite, Smoky Elestial Quartz, Smoky Quartz, Sodalite, Sphalerite, Tourmalinated Quartz, Tourmaline, Yellow Kunzite, Zeolite. *Disperse around site or between you and the site.*

– N –

Negative energy dispel: Amber, Amethyst, Black Tourmaline, Heulandite, Lapis Lazuli, Orgonite, Pollucite, Scolecite, Shungite, Smoky Quartz, Snowflake Obsidian, Sodalite, Stilbite, Thompsonite *and see Detoxification page 230*

Negative ions, increase: Amethyst, Angel's Wing Calcite, Bismuth, Germanium, Heulandite, Jasper, Klinoptilolith, Lepidolite, Orgonite, Pollucite, Quartz, Scolecite, Shungite, Sphalerite, Stilbite, Thompsonite, Tourmaline

Nuclear sites, transmute radiation effects: Amber, Aventurine, Boron, Chlorite Quartz, Colemanite, Covellite, Galena *(caution: toxic)*, Graphic Smoky Quartz, Hackmanite, Kernite, Larimar, Lepidolite, Libyan Gold Tektite, Malachite, Malacolla, Mica, Morion, Orgonite,

Rainbow Covellite, Shungite, Smoky Elestial Quartz, Smoky Quartz, Sodalite, Tantalite, Tektite, Torbernite, Velvet Malachite. *Disperse essence around site or between you and the source.*

– O –

Other people's thoughts invading: Amethyst, Auralite 23, Black Tourmaline, Fluorite, Labradorite, Shamanite. *Chakra:* third eye

– P –

Pollutants, anti: Amazonite, Amber, Aventurine, Black Tourmaline, Brown Jasper, Chlorite Quartz, Malachite, Orgonite, Purple Tourmaline, Quantum Quattro, Shieldite, Shungite, Sodalite, Turquoise. *Chakra:* earth star. *Disperse in environment.*

Protection, angelic: Amethyst, Angelite, Angel's Wing Calcite, Celestite, Selenite, Seraphinite

Protection, aura: see Aura page 108

Protection, children: Agate, Bloodstone, Blue Lace Agate, Carnelian, Green Moss Agate, Jade, Ruby, Youngite. Wear constantly.

Protection, during astral travel: Brecciated Jasper, Kyanite, Leopardskin Agate, Preseli Bluestone, Red Jasper, Shaman Quartz, Snakeskin Agate, Stibnite, Yellow Jasper *and see Shamanic journey* page 200

Protection, from crime and/or violence: Jet, Sardonyx, Selenite, Turquoise

Protection from negative energies: Amethyst, Apache

Tear, Black Kyanite, Black Obsidian, Black Onyx, Black Tourmaline, Bornite, Celestite, Chalcopyrite, Citrine, Elestial Quartz, Eye of the Storm, Flint, Jet, Kunzite, Plancheite, Quartz, Rose Quartz, Selenite, Shungite, Smoky Quartz. *Wear or grid around home or environment.*

Protection, general: Agate, Amber, Apache Tear, Aventurine, Banded Agate, Beryl, Black Kyanite, Black Obsidian, Black Tourmaline, Boji Stones, Bronzite, Calcite, Carnelian, Cat's Eye, Chalcedony, Chiastolite, Chrysoprase, Citrine, Dravide Tourmaline, Emerald, Fire Agate, Fire Opal, Flint, Fluorite, Golden Topaz, Halite, Hanksite, Heliodor (Golden Beryl), Hematite, Hematoid Quartz, Herkimer Diamond, Holey Stones, Honey Calcite, Imperial Topaz, Jade, Jasper, Jet, Labradorite, Lapis Lazuli, Lepidolite, Magnesite (Lodestone), Mahogany Obsidian, Malachite, Marble, Mookaite Jasper, Moss Agate, Nuummite, Ocean Jasper, Peridot, Petrified Wood, Polychrome Jasper, Prehnite, Pumice, Pyrite, Quartz, Red Jasper, Ruby, Rutilated Quartz, Sapphire, Sard, Sardonyx, Selenite, Serpentine, Shungite, Snowflake Obsidian, Staurolite, Sulphur, Sunstone, Tiger's Eye, Topaz, Tourmalinated Quartz, Tourmaline, Tree Agate, Turritella Agate, Turquoise, Yellow Jasper, Zircon

Protection, home, other buildings: Black Tourmaline, Dravide Tourmaline, Halite, Hanksite, Holey Stones, Malachite, Quartz, Rose Quartz, Ruby, Sardonyx, Selenite, Witches Finger

Protection, possessions: Ruby, Sardonyx, Zircon

Psychic attack, protect against: Black Tourmaline, Brandenberg Amethyst, Labradorite, Master Shamanite, Mohawkite, Nunderite, Nuummite, Polychrome Jasper, Richterite, Shungite, Tantalite, Tugtupite. (*Wear essence constantly.*) *Chakra:* throat, higher heart

Psychic overwhelm: Labradorite, Limonite, Master Shamanite

Psychic shield: Actinolite, Amphibole, Azotic Topaz, Aztee, Black Tourmaline, Bornite, Bowenite (New Jade), Brandenberg Amethyst, Brazilianite, Celestobarite, Chlorite Shaman Quartz, Crackled Fire Agate, Eye of the Storm, Fiskenaesset Ruby, Frondellite with Strengite, Gabbro, Graphic Smoky Quartz (Zebra Stone), Hanksite, Iridescent Pyrite, Keyiapo, Labradorite, Lorenzite (Ramsayite), Marcasite, Master Shamanite, Mohave Turquoise, Mohawkite, Owyhee Blue Opal, Polychrome Jasper, Purpurite, Pyromorphite, Quantum Quattro, Red Amethyst, Silver Leaf Jasper, Smoky Amethyst, Smoky Elestial Quartz, Tantalite, Thunder Egg, Valentinite and Stibnite, Xenotine

Psychic vampirism, block: Actinolite, Ammolite, Apple Aura Quartz, Banded Agate, Gaspeite, Green Aventurine, Green Fluorite, Iridescent Pyrite, Jade, Jet, Labradorite, Lemurian Aquitane Calcite, Nunderite, Prasiolite, Tantalite, Xenotine

– R –

Radiation, counteract: Aventurine, Black Tourmaline, Boron, Chlorite Quartz, Colemanite, Covellite, Galena (*caution: toxic*), Graphic Smoky Quartz, Hackmanite, Jasper, Kernite, Klinoptilolith, Kunzite, Malachite, Morion, Orgonite, Ouro Verde, Quartz, Rainbow Covellite, Reinerite, Smoky Elestial, Smoky Elestial Quartz, Smoky Quartz, Sodalite, Tantalite, Tektite, Torbernite, Uranophane, Velvet Malachite, Yellow Kunzite. *Chakra:* earth star, base. *Disperse around source.*

Radioactivity: Annabergite, Boron, Chlorite Quartz, Colemanite, Galena (*caution: toxic*), Herkimer Diamond, Kernite, Kunzite, Malachite, Orgonite, Reinerite. *Drop essence around source.*

Radon gas: Boron, Chlorite Quartz, Covellite, Danburite, Diaspore, Eye of the Storm (rough form), Graphic Smoky Quartz, Herkimer Diamond, Klinoptilolith, Libyan Gold Tektite, Malachite, Morion Quartz, Ouro Verde, Shungite, Smoky Elestial Quartz, Smoky Quartz, Sodalite, Tektite, Torbernite, Yellow Kunzite. *Disperse around source.*

Restore earth's meridians: Aragonite, Celtic Golden Healer Quartz, Rhodozite

– S –

Sick building syndrome: Black Tourmaline, Chlorite Quartz, Covellite, Galena (*caution: toxic*), Graphic Smoky Quartz, Hackmanite, Lepidolite, Marble, Morion, Orgonite, Preseli Bluestone, Quartz, Selenite, Shieldite, Shungite, Smoky Elestial Quartz, Smoky Quartz, Sodalite, Trummer Jasper. *Disperse essence around building or on anchor crystals. Or disperse or spritz around aura.*

Stagnant energy, disperse: Black Tourmaline, Calcite,

Chrome Diopside, Clear Topaz, Eye of the Storm, Garnet in Quartz, Orgonite, Poppy Jasper, Quartz, Ruby Lavender Quartz, Sedona Stone, Shaman Quartz, Shungite, Smoky Quartz, Spirit Quartz, Tantalite *and see Negative energy page 235. Chakra:* base, dantien

Study/home office: Amethyst, Ammolite, Fluorite, Jade, Pyrite, Sodalite

– T –

Toxic earth meridians: Amber, Chlorite Quartz, Granite, Graphic Smoky Quartz, Kambaba Jasper, Marble, Mohawkite, Orgonite, Preseli Bluestone, Quartz, Shieldite, Shungite, Smoky Elestial Quartz, Snakeskin Pyrite, Sodalite, Valentinite and Stibnite

Toxicity: Amber, Arsenopyrite, Champagne Aura Quartz, Chlorite Quartz, Green Jasper, Klinoptilolith, Morion Quartz, Orgonite, Rutilated Quartz, Shieldite, Smoky Elestial Quartz, Smoky Quartz, Snakeskin Pyrite, Sodalite, Sunshine Aura Quartz, Tourmalinated Quartz, Valentinite and Stibnite. *Chakra:* dantien, earth, spleen

Toxicity, disperse from environment: Chlorite Quartz, Chrysanthemum Stone, Halite, Hanksite, Orgonite, Shieldite, Shungite, Smoky Quartz, Sodalite. *Disperse essence in environment.*

– W –

War zones: Afghanite, Eye of the Storm (Judy's Jasper), Tanzanite. *Disperse around environment or on to a crystal on a map.*

Workplace harmonisers: Amber, Black Tourmaline, Clear Quartz, Eye of the Storm, Fluorite, Green Chlorite Quartz, Rose Quartz, Shungite, Siberian Green Quartz, Smoky Quartz, Turquoise

– X –

X-rays, prevent damage from: Amazonite, Black Moonstone, Chlorite Quartz, Herkimer Diamond, Lepidolite, Malachite, Malacolla, Orgonite, Shieldite, Shungite, Smoky Elestial Quartz, Smoky Herkimer, Smoky Quartz, Sodalite, Torbernite (use under supervision). *Rub crystal essence over site or around aura, take crystal essence frequently.*

Karmic, ancestral and past life essences

Personal trauma and transgenerational memories are held in the so-called 'junk DNA', affecting the karmic blueprint and our subtle energy fields. The karmic blueprint carries the impact of all our experiences from life to life in whatever dimension that they may have occurred. 'Junk DNA', the subtle blueprints and the Akashic Record are part of our inner landscape. In addition to our own personal stuff, 'junk DNA' is what gets passed down through the ancestral line so it's where we tune in to a vast field of experience much wider than our own. It is found in each cell of our bodies, so it has important implications for who you are, on many levels.

– Crystal Prescriptions volume 6

242 Crystal essences assist the subtle bodies, the chakras, DNA and the endocrine system to reprogram the past and replace old patterns with new, positive programs *even where a situation goes back to past generations.* (See 'junk DNA' below and in *Crystal Prescriptions volume 6*.) They take advantage of the brain's neuroplasticity:

The brain's ability to reorganize itself by forming new neural connections throughout life. Neuroplasticity allows the neurons (nerve cells) in the brain to compensate for injury and disease and to adjust their activities in response to new situations or to changes in their environment.

– http://www.medicinenet.com

A choice of crystal prescriptions is offered because each person's ancestral and karmic history is unique. As is the ancestral timeline. So, match crystals for the essences with your particular field energy.

Some crystals have a much finer vibration than others, working from the subtle ancestral or karmic blueprint to adjust the physical body and 'junk DNA'. Earthy, lower vibration crystals operate at the physical level first to effect permanent changes in the 'junk DNA', the cells of the physical body, and then the karmic blueprint. Other crystals operate more subtly, bringing underlying causes to the surface for resolution, so that you may need to use a series of essences sequentially or in a concatenation process (see page 70). Karmic and ancestral causes of dis-ease may overlap, and it's not unknown for a soul to reincarnate further down the ancestral line to heal an issue for the good of the whole line. Fortunately it is not necessary to have the details, simply to use the appropriate crystals to create the essence.

Karmic dis-ease

Karma is not a matter of punishment or blame but of balancing out the past and allowing the soul to evolve. Karmic dis-ease is subtle and not always related to physical illness. It occurs on physical, emotional, mental and spiritual levels and can be carried forward from previous lives or from an ancestral source. Karmic disease, based on the soul's dis-ease, arises out of wounds, injuries, attitudes and patterns such as remaining on a karmic or ancestral treadmill – 'the same old same old' – or the effects of curses carried forward from past into present via the 'etheric or karmic blueprint' that creates the new physical and subtle bodies. If the blueprint is returned to balance, the dis-ease dissipates and the transformed pattern filters down into the physical body. Karmic dis-ease may also offer an incarnating soul the opportunity to learn certain attributes: patience, tolerance, compassion etc. that the soul feels have been overlooked in other lives. Or, it may offer someone else an opportunity to grow. If this is the case, a situation is unlikely to be 'cured', but an essence may assist all the souls concerned to bring out the underlying soul learning with grace and ease. (For deeper insight, see *Crystal Prescriptions: Crystals for ancestral clearing, soul retrieval, spirit release and karmic healing. An A-Z guide. Volume 6.*)

Ancestral essences

Essences for issues that have passed forward from an ancestral source can be taken by one of the family, who acts as a surrogate for the whole line. Or, the essence can be dripped on to a crystal placed on an ancestral photograph or the family tree if one is available. One of the most potent ways of restoring balance to the family line so that the benefits radiate out into future generations is to stimulate the potential carried in the so-called 'junk DNA'. (Details and further methods of ancestral healing will be found in *Crystal Prescriptions volume 6*.)

Essences embrace both creation and evolution, assisting us to reformat our DNA into a positive mode.

A-Z Directory

Choose 1–4 crystals from an entry when creating your essence.

– A –

Abandonment: Hematite Quartz, Mangano Calcite, Rhodonite, Selenite, Tangerose, Tugtupite. *Chakra:* past life, heart

Abuse: Apricot Quartz, Aventurine, Azeztulite with Morganite, Eilat Stone, Golden Healer, Honey Opal, Lazurine, Lemurian Jade, Morganite with Azeztulite, Pink Crackle Quartz, Proustite, Red Quartz, Rhodolite Garnet, Rhodonite, Septarian, Shiva Lingam, Shiva Shell, Smoky Amethyst, Smoky Citrine, Xenotine. *Chakra:* base, sacral, three-chambered heart

Abuse, break away from: Cradle of Life (Humankind), Freedom Stone, Rhodolite Garnet, Rhodonite, Xenotine. *Chakra:* sacral and solar plexus

Abuse, clear emotional: Apricot Quartz, Aventurine, Azeztulite with Morganite, Cradle of Life (Humankind), Honey Opal, Lazurine, Mount Shasta Opal, Rose Quartz, Rosophia, Smoky Rose Quartz, Tugtupite, Xenotine. *Chakra:* sacral, heart

Abuse, sexual, heal: Apricot Quartz, Eilat Stone, Golden Healer, Proustite, Rhodolite Garnet, Rhodonite, Shiva Lingam. *Chakra:* base, sacral

Access: Brandenberg Amethyst, Cavansite, Chrysotile, Dream Quartz, Dumortierite, Faden Quartz, Fiskenaesset Ruby, Lemurian Seed, Nuummite, Oregon Opal, Preseli

Bluestone, Trigonic Quartz. *Chakra:* past life, third eye

Addiction, past life causes of: Crystal Cap Amethyst, Fenster Quartz, Kornerupine, Red Amethyst, Smoky Amethyst, Vera Cruz Amethyst. *Chakra:* past life, base *and see Addictions page 184*

Akashic Record: Afghanite, Amphibole, Andescine Labradorite, Blue Euclase, Brandenberg Amethyst, Brookite, Cathedral Quartz, Celestial Quartz, Chinese Writing Quartz, Dumortierite, Eilat Stone, Heulandite, K2, Keyiapo, Lemurian Aquitane Calcite, Merkabite Calcite, Merlinite, Phosphosiderite, Prophecy Stone, Serpentine in Obsidian, Sichuan Quartz, Tanzanite, Tremolite, Trigonic Quartz. *Chakra:* past life, third eye, crown

Ancestral attachment/myths/stories carried in the genes: Anandalite, Ancestralite, Brandenberg Amethyst, Celtic Quartz, Cradle of Life (Humankind), Datolite, Fairy Quartz, Freedom Stone, Lakelandite, Lemurian Seed, Preseli Bluestone, Rainforest Jasper, Seftonite, Smoky Elestial, Spirit Quartz. *Chakra:* soma, causal vortex, solar plexus

Ancestral healer crystals: Ammolite, Ammonite, Anandalite, Ancestral healer (large crystal with a distinctive flat pathway running up the crystal from bottom to top), Ancestralite, Brandenberg, Celtic Chevron Quartz, Chrysotile, Cradle of Life (Humankind), Dumortierite, Elestial Quartz, Fairy Quartz, Freedom Stone, Kambaba Jasper, Lakelandite, Mother and child formation (a large crystal to which is attached a smaller crystal or crystals that appears to be enfolded), Petrified Wood, Preseli Bluestone, Seftonite, Smithsonite, Smoky Elestial, Spirit Quartz, Stromatolite, Turritella Agate, Wind Fossil Agate. *Chakra:* past life, causal vortex

Ancestral issues: Ancestralite, Celtic Quartz, Cradle of Life (Humankind), Golden Healer, Lakelandite, Porphyrite (Chinese Letter Stone), Seftonite. *Chakra:* past life, causal vortex, alta major

Ancestral line, healing: Amber, Ancestralite, Brandenberg Amethyst, Candle Quartz, Chlorite Quartz, Cradle of Life (Humankind), Crinoidal Limestone, Datolite, Fairy Quartz, Golden Healer, Ilmenite, Kambaba Jasper, Lemurian Aquitane Calcite, Mohawkite, Petrified Wood, Prasiolite, Rainforest Jasper, Seftonite, Shaman Quartz, Smoky Elestial Quartz, Spirit Quartz, Stromatolite. *Chakra:* past life, base, causal vortex

Ancestral patterns: Ancestralite, Anthrophyllite, Arfvedsonite, Candle Quartz, Celadonite, Celtic Quartz, Cradle of Life (Humankind), Crinoidal Limestone, Eclipse Stone, Garnet in Quartz, Glendonite, Golden Healer, Green Ridge Quartz, Holly Agate, Lakelandite, Mohawkite, Porphyrite (Chinese Letter Stone), Prasiolite, Rainbow Covellite, Rainbow Mayanite, Scheelite, Seftonite, Shaman Quartz with Chlorite, Starseed Quartz, Wind Fossil Agate. Chakra: past life, causal vortex, alta major

Anorexia from past life causes: Ancestralite, Azotic Topaz, Cradle of Life (Humankind), Lakelandite, Mystic

Topaz, Orange Kyanite, Picasso Jasper, Tugtupite. *Chakra:* earth star, base, heart

Atlantis issues: Ajo Blue Calcite, Atlantasite, Atlantean Lovestars, Hanksite, Heulandite, Lemurian Seed, Mount Shasta Opal, Sacred Scribes. *Chakra:* past life

Authority figures, difficulties with: Ancestralite, Barite, Cradle of Life (Humankind), Freedom Stone, Gaia's Blood Flint (maternal), Lakelandite, Milky Way Quartz (paternal), Pietersite, Pyrophyllite, Sceptre Quartz, Sonora Sunrise. *Chakra:* dantien, navel

Autoimmune diseases, hereditary: Anandalite, Bastnasite, Brandenberg Amethyst, Chinese Red Quartz, Cradle of Life (Humankind), Diaspore (Zultanite), Gabbro, Golden Healer, Granite, Lakelandite, Mookaite Jasper, Paraiba Tourmaline, Quantum Quattro, Richterite, Rosophia, Shungite, Tangerose, Titanite (Sphene), Winchite. *Chakra:* dantien, higher heart

Autonomy: Candle Quartz, Carnelian, Cradle of Life (Humankind), Faden Quartz, Flint, Freedom Stone, Frondellite with Strengite, Pietersite, Pyrolusite, Pyrophyllite, Rhodolite Garnet, Ussingite. *Chakra:* dantien

– B –

Balance male/female energies: Alexandrite, Amphibole Quartz, Day and Night Quartz, Gaia's Blood and Milky Way Flint, Khutnohorite, Plinolith, Prairie Tanzanite, Shiva Lingam. *Chakra:* base and sacral

Beliefs that no longer serve, release: Ancestralite, Cradle of Life (Humankind), Freedom Stone, Geothite,

Lakelandite. *Chakra:* past life, third eye

Betrayal: Celtic Golden Healer, Golden Green Ridge Quartz, Golden Healer, Mangano Calcite, Quantum Quattro, Rhodonite, Smoky Rose Quartz, Tugtupite. *Chakra:* three-chambered heart, past life, heart, navel

Bigotry, overcome effects of: Chrysanthemum Stone, Rose Quartz, Tugtupite. *Chakra:* heart

Bitterness: Gaspeite, Hubnerite, Rose Quartz. *Chakra:* heart

Blockages from past lives: Ajo Blue Calcite, Lemurian Seed, Nuummite, Orange Kyanite, Purple Scapolite, Rainbow Mayanite, Rhodozite, Serpentine in Obsidian. *Chakra:* past life

Body, acceptance of: Candle Quartz, Eye of the Storm, Phenacite, Vanadinite. *Chakra:* earth, base, crown

Body, discomfort at being in: Candle Quartz, Pearl Spa Dolomite, Quantum Quattro, Strontianite. *Chakra:* earth star, base, sacral, dantien

Break patterns: Arfvedsonite, Celadonite, Garnet in Quartz, Green Ridge Quartz, Lemurian Seed, Owyhee Blue Opal, Porphyrite (Chinese Letter Stone), Rainbow Covellite, Rainbow Mayanite, Rhodozite, Scheelite, Stellar Beam Calcite

Broken heart: Cobalto Calcite, Mangano Vesuvianite, Tugtupite. *Chakra:* past life, heart

– C –

Causal vortex chakra: see page 111

Causes of disease in the karmic or ancestral line,

discover: Ammolite, Ancestralite, Chrysotile, Cradle of Life (Humankind), crystal from ancestral or past life locality, Faden Quartz, Golden Healer, Indicolite Quartz, Kambaba Jasper, Lakelandite, Petrified Wood, Pholocomite, Preseli Bluestone, Seftonite, Stromatolite. *Chakra:* past life, causal vortex, earth star

    anxiety or fear: Candle Quartz, Dumortierite, Eilat Stone, Khutnohorite, Oceanite, Rose Quartz, Tangerose, Thunder Egg, Tremolite, Tugtupite. *Chakra:* solar plexus, causal vortex, past life

    damaged immune system passing down: Ancestralite, Blizzard Stone, Brandenberg Amethyst, Celtic Quartz, Cradle of Life (Humankind), Diaspore (Zultanite), Gabbro, Golden Healer, Lakelandite, Lemurian Jade, Mookaite Jasper, Nzuri Moyo, Ocean Blue Jasper, Pyrite and Sphalerite, Quantum Quattro, Que Sera, Schalenblende, Shungite, Stone of Solidarity, Super 7, Tangerose, Titanite (Sphene), Winchite. *Chakra:* dantien, higher heart, causal vortex, past life

    emotional exhaustion from over-caring for family: Candle Quartz, Cradle of Life (Humankind), Golden Healer, Mount Shasta Opal, Prehnite with Epidote, Rose Quartz. *Chakra:* solar plexus

    emotional wounds: Ajoite, Bustamite, Cassiterite, Cobalto Calcite, Eilat Stone, Gaia Stone, Golden Healer, Macedonian Opal, Mookaite Jasper, Orange River Quartz, Piemontite, Rathbunite™, Rhodonite, Rose Quartz, Turquoise, Xenotine. *Chakra:* higher heart

mental stress: Candle Quartz, Eye of the Storm, Guinea Fowl Jasper, Lemurian Gold Opal, Richterite, Shungite. *Chakra:* third eye, soma

negative attitudes or emotions: Ancestralite, Candle Quartz, Kornerupine, Pyrite in Quartz, Thunder Egg. *Chakra:* three-chambered heart, crown

past life wounds: Ajo Quartz, Ajoite, Anandalite, Ancestralite, Celtic Quartz, Golden Healer, Green Ridge Quartz, Lakelandite, Lemurian Seed, Macedonian Opal, Mookaite Jasper, Rathbunite™, Rosophia, Scheelite, Xenotine. *Chakra:* past life, causal vortex, earth star

shock, trauma or psychic attack: Apricot Quartz, Black Tourmaline, Empowerite, Golden Healer, Guardian Stone, Linerite, Mohave Turquoise, Mohawkite, Oceanite, Polychrome Jasper, Richterite, Ruby Lavender Quartz, Shungite, Tantalite, Victorite

Celibacy, reverse vow of: Anandalite™, Citrine, Dragon Stone, Freedom Stone, Kundalini Quartz, Serpentine in Obsidian, Shiva Lingam, Smoky Citrine, Triplite. *Chakra:* base, sacral, causal vortex

Cellular matrix: Ancestralite, Brandenberg Amethyst, Cradle of Life (Humankind), Eye of the Storm, Gold in Quartz, Golden Healer, Kambaba Jasper, Mangano Vesuvianite, Rainbow Mayanite, Rosophia, Shungite, Stromatolite, Terralimunite. *Chakra:* higher heart, alta major

Cellular memory: Ajo Quartz, Ajoite, Ancestralite, Andean Blue Opal, Azotic Topaz, Brandenberg

Amethyst, Bustamite, Celtic Quartz, Chrysotile, Cradle of
Life (Humankind), Datolite, Dumortierite, Eilat Stone,
Elestial Quartz, Eye of the Storm, Golden Healer,
Heulandite, Kambaba Jasper, Leopardskin Jasper,
Lepidocrosite, Nuummite, Preseli Bluestone, Rainbow
Mayanite, Rhodozite, Sichuan Quartz, Smoky Quartz
with Aegerine, Sodalite, Spirit Quartz, Stromatolite,
Valentinite and Stibnite. *Chakra:* dantien, alta major,
causal vortex

Chastity, previous vow of: Kundalini Quartz, Menalite,
Smoky Citrine. *Chakra:* past life, base, sacral

Conflict: Bixbite, Champagne Aura Quartz, Fluorapatite,
Purpurite, Rainbow Mayanite, Trigonic Quartz

Contracts, renegotiate: Anandalite, Ancestralite, Boli
Stone, Cradle of Life (Humankind), Dumortierite,
Freedom Stone, Gabbro, Nuummite, Prasiolite, Purple
Scapolite, Quantum Quattro, Red Amethyst, Shiva
Lingam. *Chakra:* past life, alta major, causal vortex

Control freak: Chrysotile, Freedom Stone, Ice Quartz,
Lazulite, Lemurian Aquitane Calcite, Spiders Web
Obsidian. *Chakra:* dantien

Curses, break ancestral: Freedom Stone, Nuummite,
Purpurite, Quantum Quattro, Shattuckite, Stibnite,
Tiger's Eye, Tourmalinated Quartz. *Chakra:* past life,
throat, third eye, causal vortex

– D –

Death, unhealed trauma: Blue Euclase, Brandenberg,
Cavansite, Gaia Stone, Green Ridge Quartz, Lemurian

Jade, Lemurian Seed, Oceanite, Quantum Quattro, Sea Sediment Jasper, Smoky Elestial Quartz, Spirit Quartz, Tantalite, Victorite. *Chakra:* past life, earth star, base, heart
Debts, recognise: Lemurian Seed, Nuummite, Purple Scapolite. *Chakra:* past life, solar plexus
Dis-ease: Dumortierite, Lemurian Seed, Sichuan Quartz. *Chakra:* past life

– E –

Emotional ancestral trauma: Ancestral country/state stone, Ajo Blue Calcite, Ajoite, Ancestralite, Blue Euclase, Cavansite, Cobalto Calcite, Empowerite, Epidote, Gaia Stone, Golden Healer, Graphic Smoky Quartz, Guinea Fowl Jasper, Holly Agate, Kambaba Jasper, Mangano Vesuvianite, Oceanite, Orange River Quartz, Oregon Opal, Peanut Wood, Petrified Wood, Porcelain Jasper, Ruby Lavender Quartz, Sea Sediment Jasper, Seftonite, Stromatolite, Tantalite, Tugtupite, Victorite. *Chakra:* solar plexus, past life

Emotional attachments: Aegirine, Drusy Golden Healer, Ilmenite, Novaculite, Nuummite, Rainbow Mayanite, Smoky Amethyst, Stibnite, Tantalite, Tinguaite. *Chakra:* past life

Emotional blockages from past lives: Aegirine, Datolite, Dumortierite, Frondellite plus Strengite, Graphic Smoky Quartz (Zebra Stone), Prehnite with Epidote, Pyrite and Sphalerite, Quantum Quattro, Rainbow Obsidian, Rhodolite Garnet, Rhodozite, Rose Elestial Quartz, Serpentine in Obsidian, Tugtupite. *Chakra:* past life, three-chambered heart, causal vortex *and see Healing page 257*

Emotional body: Oregon Opal *and see page 250*

Emotional healing: Boli Stone, Cobalto Calcite, Mangano Vesuvianite, Orange Sphalerite, Prairie Tanzanite, Shungite

Emotional hooks: Drusy Golden Healer, Geothite, Nunderite, Orange Kyanite, Pyromorphite, Tantalite

Emotional manipulation: Pink Lemurian Seed, Rhodolite Garnet, Tantalite. *Chakra:* sacral, solar plexus, third eye, spleen

Emotional pain: Blue Euclase, Cobalto Calcite. *Chakra:* past life, heart, higher heart, solar plexus

Emotional trauma: Ajo Blue Calcite, Blue Euclase, Cavansite, Gaia Stone, Guinea Fowl Jasper, Holly Agate, Mangano Vesuvianite, Oceanite, Oregon Opal, Peanut Wood, Ruby Lavender Quartz, Sea Sediment Jasper, Tantalite, Victorite

Emotional wounds: Ajo Quartz, Eudialyte, Fiskenaesset Ruby, Macedonian Opal, Moldau Quartz, Mookaite Jasper, Prehnite with Epidote, Rathbunite™, Rosophia, Scheelite, Tangerose, Tugtupite, Xenotine. *Chakra:* past life, heart, higher heart, solar plexus

Entity attachment: Chrysotile in Serpentine, Drusy Golden Healer, Ilmenite, Larvikite, Lemurian Aquitane Calcite, Novaculite, Nuummite, Pyromorphite, Quantum Quattro, Rainbow Mayanite, Stibnite, Tantalite, Tinguaite, Tugtupite, Valentinite and Stibnite. *Chakra:* past life, sacral, solar plexus, spleen, third eye

Ethnic conflict: Afghanite, Ancestralite, Azeztulite with Morganite, Catlinite, Champagne Aura Quartz, Chinese Red Quartz, Eye of the Storm, Fluorapatite, Trigonic Quartz, Tugtupite. *Disperse around aura and site of conflict or on a map.*

— F —

Family patterns: Arfvedsonite, Brandenberg Amethyst, Celadonite, Dumortierite, Fenster Quartz, Garnet in Quartz, Polychrome Jasper, Porphyrite (Chinese Letter Stone), Rainbow Covellite, Scheelite. *Chakra:* past life, sacral

Family scapegoat: Ancestralite, Blue Lace Agate, Celtic Chevron Quartz, Celtic Golden Healer, Green Tourmaline, Larimar, Ocean Jasper, Rose Quartz, Scapolite, Tree Agate. *Chakra:* causal vortex, base

Fear, irrational from past lives: Amethyst, Cradle of Life (Humanity), Eye of the Storm, Revelation Stone

Fear of abandonment or rejection: Clevelandite, Rhodolite Garnet, Rhodozaz, Rose Quartz

Fear of death: Arsenopyrite, Ruby in Kyanite, Ruby in Zoisite, Selenite

Fear of dirt and bacteria: Frondellite, Shungite

Fear of failure: Avalonite, Elestial Quartz

Fear of responsibility: Brazilianite, Hemimorphite, Ocean Jasper, Paraiba Tourmaline, Quantum Quattro

Fear of the unknown: Bastnasite

– G –

Genocide: Ancestralite, Catlinite, Cradle of Life (Humankind), Freedom Stone, Morion Quartz, Trigonic Quartz. *Chakra:* earth star and Gaia gateway. *Disperse around site or on a map.*

Grief, unhealed: Empowerite, Mangano Vesuvianite, Oregon Opal, Tugtupite, Voegesite. *Chakra:* past life, heart

– H –

Healing: Blizzard Stone, Chinese Red Quartz, Dumortierite, Garnet in Quartz, Lodalite, Oregon Opal, Peanut Wood, Picasso Jasper, Seftonite, Serpentine in Obsidian, Tanzanite, Tibetan Quartz, Tugtupite, Voegesite. *Chakra:* past life

Heart pain/heartbreak: Blue Euclase, Brandenberg Amethyst, Cobalto Calcite, Mangano Vesuvianite, Tugtupite. *Chakra:* past life, higher heart

Hyperactivity due to effects of: Dianite, Yellow Scapolite. *Chakra:* past life, third eye

– I –

Imperatives: Ammolite, Lemurian Aquitane Calcite, Novaculite, Tantalite

Implants: Amechlorite, Cryolite, Drusy Golden Healer, Holly Agate, Ilmenite, Lemurian Aquitane Calcite, Novaculite, Nuummite, Rainbow Mayanite, Tantalite, Tinguaite

Incest, overcome effects: Cobalto Calcite, Eilat Stone,

Golden Healer, Rhodolite Garnet, Tugtupite. *Chakra:* base, sacral, solar plexus. Or spritz around aura.

Injuries: Brandenberg Amethyst, Cradle of Life, Flint. *Chakra:* past life

– J –

Jealousy: Eclipse Stone, Green Aventurine, Heulandite, Mangano Calcite, Peridot, Rainbow Mayanite, Rose Quartz, Rosophia, Tugtupite, Zircon. *Chakra:* heart

'Junk DNA', switch on potential: Anandalite, Ancestralite, Azeztulite, Cradle of Life (Humankind), Eye of the Storm, Feather Pyrite, Kambaba Jasper, Poppy Jasper, Rainbow Mayanite, Rhodozite, Stromatolite, Titanite, Trigonic Quartz. *Chakra:* causal vortex, soma, past life, dantien

– L –

Learning from past: Chrysotile, Cradle of Life (Humanity), Dumortierite. *Chakra:* past life

Lemurian issues: Ajo Blue Calcite, Dreamsicle Lemurian, Healer's Gold, Larimar, Lemurian Blue Calcite, Lemurian Jade, Lemurian Seed, Mount Shasta Opal, Sedona Stone, Selenite, Trigonic Quartz. *Chakra:* causal vortex, alta major, past life, heart seed

– M –

Manipulation: Nuummite, Tantalite

Matriarchy/mother issues: Jade, Jasper, Menalite, Shiva Lingam, Spirit Quartz. *Chakra:* navel (tummy button) *and*

see Parents

Memories: Dream Quartz, Seftonite

Mental abuse: Apricot Quartz, Golden Healer, Lazurine, Proustite, Rhodolite Garnet, Tugtupite with Nuummite, Yellow Crackle Quartz, Xenotine

Mental imperatives, release: Golden Danburite, Nuummite, Septarian, Tantalite. *Chakra:* past life

Misuse of power: Nuummite, Ocean Jasper, Smoky Lemurian Seed

– N –

Navel: see page 121

Nurturing, overcome lack of: Amblygonite, Bornite on Silver, Calcite Fairy Stone, Clevelandite, Cobalto Calcite, Drusy Blue Quartz, Flint, Golden Healer, Lazurine, Menalite, Mount Shasta Opal, Ocean Jasper, Prasiolite, Rose Quartz, Ruby Lavender Quartz, Septarian, Super 7, Tree Agate, Tugtupite. *Chakra:* higher heart, base

– P –

Parents: *Chakra:* dantien, navel (tummy button), base and sacral

> **father:** Citrine, Green Tourmaline, Jasper, Mentor formation, Milky Way Flint, Pietersite, Sunstone
>
> **mother:** Gaia's Blood Flint, Larimar, Lemurian Jade, Menalite, Moonstone, Mother and child formation, Picture Jasper, Rhodochrosite, Rose Quartz, Selenite
>
> **integrate the inner parents:** Day and Night Quartz, Shiva Lingam

And see Matriarchy/mother issues and Patriarchy/father issues.

Past life chakras: see page 119

Past, release from: Dumortierite, Elestial Quartz, Smoky Amethyst *and see Blockages from past lives above. Chakra:* past life, earth star, base

Patriarchy/father issues: Flint, Galena, Milky Way Flint, Petrified Wood, Shiva Lingam, Smoky Quartz, Stibnite, Sunstone. *Chakra:* dantien, sacral

People-pleaser, release: Anthrophyllite. *Chakra:* dantien

Persecution: Aragonite, Rose Quartz, Wulfenite. *Chakra:* past life

Phobias resulting from: Carolite, Dumortierite, Oceanite, Serpentine in Obsidian. *Chakra:* past life

Pollutants: Diaspore (Zultanite), Paraiba Tourmaline, Phlogopite, Pyrite and Sphalerite, Pyromorphite, Shungite

Psychosexual problems resulting from past: Cobalto Calcite, Dumortierite, Serpentine in Obsidian. *Chakra:* past life, base, sacral

– R –

Recall: Dumortierite, Preseli Bluestone, Revelation Stone. *Chakra:* past life, third eye

Reclaim power: Brandenberg Amethyst, Eilat Stone, Empowerite, Leopardskin Jasper, Nuummite, Owyhee Blue Opal, Rainbow Mayanite, Smoky Elestial Quartz, Tinguaite. *Chakra:* past life, base

Reconciliation: Afghanite, Chinese Red Quartz, Pink

Lazurine, Rose Quartz, Ruby Lavender Quartz. *Chakra:* heart seed

Regression: Chrysotile, Dumortierite, Preseli Bluestone, Wind Fossil Agate. *Chakra:* past life, third eye

Rejection: Cassiterite. *Chakra:* past life, heart

Releasing vows: Nuummite, Rainbow Mayanite, Stibnite, Wind Fossil Agate. *Chakra:* past life, third eye

Reprogram past patterns in hippocampus: Fluorapatite, Preseli Bluestone

Resentment: Eclipse Stone, Tugtupite. *Chakra:* past life, base

Restraint, psychological, emotional or mental: Libyan Gold Tektite, Tugtupite. *Chakra:* past life, heart

Retrieve soul parts left at previous death: Lemurian Seed, Selenite, Smoky Spirit Quartz. *Chakra:* causal vortex, past life

– S –

Sexual problems arising from past life: Eilat Stone, Rutile. *Chakra:* past life, base, sacral

Slavery, release from: Apache Tear, Freedom Stone, Malachite, Rainbow Obsidian, Rutilated Quartz, Snowflake Obsidian

Soul agreements, recognition and renegotiation: Brandenberg Amethyst, Green Ridge Quartz, Nuummite, Trigonic Quartz, Wind Fossil Agate. *Chakra:* past life, higher crown

Soul loss resulting from past: Chrysotile in Serpentine, Fulgarite

– T –

Thought forms, release: Aegirine, Pyromorphite, Scolecite, Septarian, Spectrolite, Xenotine. *Chakra:* past life, third eye

Tie cutting: Flint, Novaculite, Nuummite, Rainbow Mayanite, Smoky Amethyst. *Chakra:* past life, base, sacral, solar plexus, third eye

Trauma: Blue Euclase, Brandenberg Amethyst, Dumortierite, Empowerite, Mangano Vesuvianite, Oceanite, Oregon Opal, Red Phantom Quartz, Ruby Lavender Quartz, Smoky Elestial Quartz, Smoky Herkimer, Tantalite, Victorite

– V –

Vampirism of heart energy: Gaspeite, Greenlandite, Iridescent Pyrite, Lemurian Aquitane Calcite, Nunderite, Tantalite, Xenotine. *Chakra:* solar plexus, heart, higher heart

Vampirism of spleen energy: Gaspeite, Iridescent Pyrite, Nunderite, Tantalite, Xenotine. *Chakra:* spleen

Vows, release: Andean Opal, Dumortierite, Libyan Gold Tektite, Nuummite, Rainbow Mayanite. *Chakra:* past life

– W –

Wound imprints in etheric body: Ajo Quartz, Brandenberg Amethyst, Diaspore (Zultanite), Ethiopian Opal, Eye of the Storm, Flint, Green Ridge Quartz, Lemurian Aquitane Calcite, Lemurian Seed, Macedonian Opal, Master Shamanite, Mookaite Jasper, Rainbow

Mayanite, Seftonite, Snakeskin Pyrite, Stibnite, Tantalite. *Chakra:* past life, causal vortex. *Or rub over site.*

– Z –

Zygote damaged: Ancestralite, Brandenberg Amethyst, Celtic Chevron Quartz, Cradle of Life (Humankind), Menalite. *Chakra:* causal vortex

Physiological essences

Crystal essences have an important role to play in preventing dis-ease and keeping you healthy. They support the organs, endocrine and physiological processes in the body. And, if you do succumb to illness, they are a gentle but effective healing tool. Healing does not necessarily imply a cure, although it frequently ameliorates conditions. Crystal essences are a gentle and non-invasive process that creates balance on all levels interacting with the human energy field to heal, calm, stimulate or adjust the energies within it and to bring the body back into balance.

Choose 1–4 crystals from an entry when creating your essence.

A-Z Directory

– A –

Adrenals: see Stress and PTSD

– B –

Blood sugar imbalances: Astraline, Chinese Chromium Quartz, Chrome Diopside, Citrine, Green Shaman Quartz, Hubnerite, Malacholla, Maw Sit Sit, Mtrolite, Muscovite, Orange Kyanite, Owyhee Blue Opal, Peridot, Pink Opal, Pink Sunstone, Rose Quartz, Serpentine in Obsidian, Shungite, Sodalite, Stichtite and Serpentine, Tugtupite *and see Diabetes page 269 and Pancreas page 281. Chakra:* spleen, dantien, heart

Brain: Amber, Amethyst, Beryl, Botswana Agate, Brandenberg Amethyst, Carnelian, Crystal Cap Amethyst, Epidote, Green Tourmaline, Kyanite, Labradorite, Magnesite, Nuummite, Prehnite with Epidote, Pyrite and Sphalerite, Royal Sapphire, Schalenblende, Sodalite, Staurolite, Trigonic Quartz, Vera Cruz Amethyst, White Heulandite. *Chakra:* third eye, soma, crown, alta major

Brain, balance left-right hemispheres: Calcite, Crystal Cap Amethyst, Cumberlandite, Eudialyte, Eye of the Storm, Fluorite, Hematite with Rutile, Lilac Quartz, Rhodozite, Sodalite, Stromatolite, Sugilite, Trigonic Quartz. *Chakra:* soma

Brain, benign tumours: Natrolite and Scolecite

Brain blood flow, improve: Iron Pyrite

Brain chemistry: Barite, Stichtite

Brain damage: Amphibole, Anthrophyllite, Brandenberg Amethyst, Galaxyite, Herderite

Brain degeneration: Anthrophyllite, Sodalite

Brain detox: Amechlorite, Chlorite Quartz, Eye of the Storm, Klinoptilolith, Lapis Lazuli, Larvikite, Nuummite, Rainbow Covellite, Rhodozite, Richterite, Ruby, Shungite, Smoky Quartz with Aegerine, Sodalite, Thulite, Zircon

Brain disorders: Brandenberg Amethyst, Chalcopyrite, Galaxyite, Holly Agate, Khutnohorite, Sapphire, Sodalite, Stilbite

Brain dysfunction: Anthrophyllite, Blue Holly Agate, Cryolite, Cumberlandite, Sodalite

Brain fatigue: Apricot Quartz, Pyrite in Quartz, Strawberry Lemurian, Turquoise

Brain function: Cryolite, Phantom Calcite, Rhodozite

Brain, neural pathways: Anglesite, Celestobarite, Crystal Cap Amethyst, Feather Calcite, Feather Pyrite, Holly Agate, Larvikite, Phantom Calcite, Pyrite and Sphalerite, Schalenblende, Scolecite, Stichtite

Brain stem: Blue Moonstone, Chrysotile, Chrysotile in Serpentine, Cradle of Life, Eye of the Storm, Kambaba Jasper, Schalenblende, Stromatolite

Brain synapses: Azurite

Brain tumour: Champagne Aura Quartz, Eilat Stone, Emerald, Klinoptilolith, Nuummite, Ouro Verde

Cellular metabolism: Ammolite, Brandenberg Amethyst, Golden Healer, Pyrite in Magnesite, Sardonyx, Shungite, Tangerine Sun Aura Quartz. *Chakra:* higher heart, causal vortex, alta major

Central nervous system: Anandalite™, Anglesite, Cradle of Life (Humankind), Golden Healer, Larvikite, Merlinite, Natrolite with Scolecite, Prehnite with Epidote. *Chakra:* dantien. Or spritz around aura.

Chest: Hiddenite, Larimar, Prehnite, Quantum Quattro. *Chakra:* heart

Chromosome damage: Ancestralite, Brandenberg Amethyst, Cradle of Life (Humankind), Golden Healer, Merlinite, Stromatolite. *Chakra:* dantien, alta major

Chronic conditions: Apricot Quartz, Bismuth, Diopside

Chronic disease: Apricot Quartz, Bismuth, Cathedral Quartz, Lemurian Jade, Orgonite, Petrified Wood, Quantum Quattro, Que Sera, Shungite, Witches Finger. *Chakra:* dantien

Chronic exhaustion: Apricot Quartz, Bismuth, Bronzite, Cinnabar in Jasper, Eye of the Storm, Poppy Jasper, Prehnite with Epidote, Triplite, Trummer Jasper. *Chakra:* dantien, higher heart

Chronic fatigue syndrome: Adamite, Amethyst, Ametrine, Apricot Quartz, Aquamarine, Aragonite, Barite, Chrysotile in Serpentine, Citrine, Green Tourmaline, Orange Calcite, Petrified Wood, Pyrite in Quartz, Quartz, Rhodochrosite, Ruby, Shungite, Tourmaline, Triplite, Trummer Jasper, Zincite. *Chakra:*

dantien *and see M.E.*

Chronic illness: Cat's Eye, Danburite, Dendritic Chalcedony, Golden Danburite, Petrified Wood, Poppy Jasper, Que Sera, Shungite, Trummer Jasper. *Chakra:* earth star, solar plexus, higher heart

Circulation: Alabaster, Anglesite, Azurite and Malachite, Bloodstone, Blue Tiger's Eye, Brazilianite, Brookite, Budd Stone (African Jade), Bustamite, Candle Quartz, Citrine, Clinohumite, Dendritic Agate, Fiskenaesset Ruby, Fulgarite, Garnet in Quartz, Green Diopside, Howlite, Merlinite, Molybdenite, Morion, Ocean Jasper, Ouro Verde, Pyroxmangite, Rhodochrosite, Riebekite with Sugilite and Bustamite, Rose Quartz, Rosophia, Ruby, Stibnite, Thulite, Trigonic Quartz, Yellow Topaz. *Chakra:* dantien, heart

Circulation, defective: Blue John, Diamond, Garnet, Merlinite, Ruby, Triplite

Circulation, fortifying: Blue Herkimer with Boulangerite, Pyrope Garnet, Tanzine Aura Quartz

Circulation, peripheral: Dianite, Ouro Verde, Spangolite

Circulatory disorders: Bloodstone, Electric-blue Obsidian, Fulgarite, Hawk's Eye, Hematite, Ruby

Circulatory system: Amethyst, Bloodstone, Chalcedony, Dendritic Agate, Hematite, Iron Pyrite, Jasper, Magnetite (Lodestone), Red Jasper

Cognitive disorders: Auralite 23, Crystal Cap Amethyst, Fluorite, Golden Healer, Rhodolite Garnet, Sugilite, *and see Mind etc. page 213. Chakra:* alta major

– D –

Diabetes: see blood sugar imbalances page 265

Diabetes, eyes, oversensitive: Aquamarine, Blue Calcite, Blue Tourmaline, Celestite, Emerald, Malachite, Vivianite

DNA: Ammolite, Ancestralite, Cradle of Life (Humankind), Datolite, Eye of the Storm, Icicle Calcite, Kambaba Jasper, Lakelandite, Petrified Wood, Pyrite in Quartz, Snakeskin Pyrite, Stromatolite. *Chakra:* dantien, higher heart, past life, alta major, causal vortex

DNA degeneration, reverse: Ancestralite, Cavansite, Cradle of Life (Humankind), Eye of the Storm, Golden Healer, Natrolite with Scholecite, Petrified Wood, Pyrite in Quartz, Snakeskin Pyrite

DNA mitochondrial: Ammolite, Ancestralite, Calcite Fairy Stone, Cradle of Life (Humankind), Eye of the Storm, Feather Pyrite, Lakelandite, Menalite, Poppy Jasper, Titanite (Sphene). *Chakra:* dantien

DNA repair: Ancestralite, Brandenberg Amethyst, Cradle of Humankind, Eye of the Storm, Lakelandite, Shungite, Snakeskin Pyrite

DNA 12 strand: Ammolite, Ancestralite, Cradle of Life (Humankind), Eye of the Storm, Leopardskin Jasper, Petrified Wood, Quantum Quattro

– E –

Endocrine system: Adamite, Alexandrite, Amber, Amechlorite, Amethyst, Aquamarine, Azeztulite with Morganite, Black Moonstone, Bloodstone, Blue Quartz, Bustamite, Champagne Aura Quartz, Chrysoberyl,

Citrine, Fire Agate, Fire and Ice Quartz, Golden Healer, Golden Topaz, Green Calcite, Green Obsidian, Howlite, Magnetite, Menalite, Pargasite, Pentagonite, Peridot, Picrolite, Pietersite, Pink Heulandite, Pink Tourmaline, Poppy Jasper, Quantum Quattro, Que Sera, Rhodochrosite, Richterite, Ruby Aura Quartz, Seriphos Quartz, Smoky Amethyst, Sodalite, Topaz, Tourmaline, Trummer Jasper, Yellow Jasper. *Chakra:* dantien, higher heart

– H –

Heart: Adamite, Andean Blue Opal, Blue or Green Aventurine, Brandenberg Amethyst, Bustamite, Cacoxenite, Candle Quartz, Fiskenaesset Ruby, Garnet, Garnet in Quartz, Golden Danburite, Green Diopside, Green Heulandite, Green Obsidian, Holly Agate, Khutnohorite, Merlinite, Peridot, Picrolite, Pink or Watermelon Tourmaline, Prasiolite, Quantum Quattro, Rhodochrosite, Rhodonite, Rose Elestial Quartz, Rose Quartz, Rosophia, Sapphire, Tugtupite *and see Heart chakra page 115. Chakra:* heart

Heart attacks: Aventurine, Dioptase, Gaspeite, Tantalite, Tugtupite

Heart beat, irregular: Dumortierite, Jade, Rhodochrosite

Heart burn: Carnelian, Dioptase, Emerald, Montebrasite, Peridot, Pyrope Garnet, Pyrophyllite, Quartz

Heart chakra: see Heart chakras pages 115–117

Heart disease: Carnelian, Eudialyte, Hemimorphite, Morganite, Red Jasper, Rhodochrosite, Rhodonite, Ruby,

Smoky Amethyst, Tourmalinated Quartz, Tugtupite

Heart failure: Scheelite

Heart healer: Azeztulite with Morganite, Khutnohorite, Pyroxmangite, Rhodozaz, Roselite, Rosophia

Heart, inflammation: Blue Euclase, Hematite, Pink Lemurian Seed, Rhodozite, Sulphur in Quartz, Zoisite

Heart, invigorate: Chohua Jasper, Green Garnet, Lemurian Jade

Heart muscle: Kunzite, Septarian

Heart rhythm, disturbed: Brandenberg Amethyst, Honey Calcite, Serpentine

Heart, strengthen: Calcite, Chohua Jasper, Danburite, Erythrite, Honey Calcite, Lemurian Jade, Pink Lemurian Seed, Rose Quartz, Strawberry Quartz, Tugtupite

Heart trauma, heal: Azeztulite with Morganite, Blue Euclase, Cobalto Calcite, Gaia Stone, Larimar, Mangano Vesuvianite, Oceanite, Peanut Wood, Quantum Quattro, Rose Elestial Quartz, Roselite, Ruby Lavender Quartz, Tantalite, Victorite

Heart, unblock: Dioptase, Gaspeite, Pink Lemurian Seed, Prasiolite, Rose Quartz, Smoky Rose Quartz

Hippocampus, reset: Apatite, Blue Kyanite, Blue Moonstone, Celtic Chevron Quartz, Chevron Amethyst, Fluorapatite, K2, Magnetite, Nunderite, Porcelain Jasper, Preseli Bluestone, Tremolite, Zircon. *Disperse in the hollow halfway up back of skull just above bony ridge.*

Hormone, boost: Amechlorite, Amethyst, Cassiterite, Lepidolite, Menalite, Paraiba Tourmaline, Pietersite, Smoky Amethyst. *Chakra:* third eye, higher heart

Hormone imbalances: Amechlorite, Astrophyllite, Black Moonstone, Champagne Aura Quartz, Chinese Chromium Quartz, Chrysoprase, Citrine, Diopside, Hemimorphite, Labradorite, Menalite, Moonstone, Paraiba Tourmaline, Sonora Sunrise, Tanzine Aura Quartz, Tugtupite. *Chakra:* third eye, higher heart

Hormones, regulate: Champagne Aura Quartz, Chinese Chromium Quartz, Menalite, Smoky Amethyst, Tugtupite, Watermelon Tourmaline. *Chakra:* brow, higher heart

– I –

Immune system: see Stress and EMFs

Impotence: Basalt, Bastnasite, Carnelian, Cinnabar in Jasper, Garnet, Kundalini Quartz, Menalite, Morganite, Orange Kyanite, Poppy Jasper, Rhodonite, Shiva Lingam, Sodalite, Triplite, Variscite. *Chakra:* base, sacral, dantien

Infertility: Banded Agate, Bastnasite, Bixbite, Blue Euclase, Brookite, 'Citrine' Herkimer, Fiskenaesset Ruby, Granite, Menalite, Shiva Lingam, Spirit Quartz, Tugtupite. *Chakra:* sacral

Insulin regulation: Ammolite, Astraline, Candle Quartz, Chrysocolla, Malacholla, Maw Sit Sit, Nuummite, Pink Opal, Red Serpentine, Schalenblende, Septarian, Serpentine in Obsidian, Shungite *and see Blood sugar imbalances page 265 and Pancreas page 281. Chakra:* spleen, dantien, third eye, crown

Intercellular blockages: Fulgarite, Gold in Quartz, Golden Healer Quartz, Plancheite, Pyrite and Sphalerite,

Rhodozite, Serpentine in Obsidian

Intercellular structures: Ajo Blue Calcite, Candle Quartz, Cradle of Life, Gold in Quartz, Golden Healer Quartz, Lemurian Aquitane Calcite, Messina Quartz, Quantum Quattro, Que Sera, Pollucite, Rhodozite, Septarian

Intestinal disorders: Bastnasite, Bismuth, Brown Tourmaline, Cryolite, Gaspeite, Halite, Hanksite, Honey Calcite, Orange Calcite, Scolecite, Septarian. *Chakra:* sacral, dantien

Irritable bowel syndrome (IBS): Amblygonite, Bastnasite, Calcite, Cryolite, Montebrasite, Pumice, Rosophia, Scolecite, Xenotine. *Chakra:* dantien

– J –

Joints: Azurite, Calcite, Cat's Eye Quartz, Dioptase, Hematite, Magnetite (Lodestone), Messina Quartz, Petrified Wood, Phantom Calcite, Poldarvarite, Rhodonite, Rhodozite

Joints, calcified: Calcite, Calcite Fairy Stone, Dinosaur Bone

Joints, flexibility: Bastnasite, Cavansite, Kimberlite, Peach Selenite, Prehnite with Epidote, Selenite Phantom, Strontianite

Joints, inflammation: Hematite, Hematite with Malachite, Lapis Lazuli, Malachite, Nzuri Moyo, Peach Selenite, Rhodonite, Rhodozite, Shungite, Sulphur in Quartz

Joints, mobilize: Aztee, Calcite Fairy Stone, Fluorite, Nzuri Moyo, Petrified Wood, Prehnite with Epidote, Red

Calcite, Strontianite

Joints, pain: Blue Euclase, Cathedral Quartz, Champagne Aura Quartz, Eilat Stone, Flint, Khutnohorite, Nzuri Moyo, Quantum Quattro, Rhodozite, Tantalite

Joints, problems: Amber, Apatite, Fluorite, Lepidolite, Obsidian, Sulphur (*caution: toxic*)

Joints, strengthening: Aragonite, Calcite, Clevelandite, Dinosaur Bone, Tantalite

Joints, swollen: Malachite, Nzuri Moyo, Shungite, Trigonic Quartz

– K –

Kidney degeneration: Honey Calcite, Quantum Quattro, Quartz, Red Jasper, Rosophia, Yellow Jasper

Kidney stones: Jasper, Magnesite, Rhyolite. Mix essence with apple juice and olive oil.

Kidneys: Amber, Aquamarine, Bastnasite, Beryl, Black Moonstone, Bloodstone, Blue Quartz, Brookite, Carnelian, Chohua Jasper, Chrysocolla, Citrine, Conichalcite, Diopside, Fiskenaesset Ruby, Gaspeite, Hematite, Heulandite, Jade, Jadeite, Leopardskin Jasper, Libyan Gold Tektite, Muscovite, Nephrite, Nunderite, Nuummite, Orange Calcite, Prehnite with Epidote, Quantum Quattro, Rhodochrosite, Rose or Smoky Quartz, Rosophia, Septarian, Serpentine, Serpentine in Obsidian, Shungite, Sonora Sunrise, Stromatolite, Tanzanite, Topaz. *Chakra:* dantien, solar plexus. *Rub over kidneys.*

Kidneys, cleanse: Atacamite, Bloodstone, Brazilianite,

Eye of the Storm (Judy's Jasper), Fire and Ice Quartz, Hematite, Jade, Klinoptilolith, Nephrite, Nuummite, Opal, Prehnite with Epidote, Red or Yellow Jasper, Rose Quartz

Kidneys, detoxify: Amechlorite, Chlorite Quartz, Chohua Jasper, Chrysocolla, Eye of the Storm, Fire and Ice Quartz, Fiskenaesset Ruby, Kambaba Jasper, Klinoptilolith, Larvikite, Leopardskin Jasper, Nuummite, Pyrite in Magnesite, Quantum Quattro, Rainbow Covellite, Richterite, Seraphinite, Shungite, Smoky Quartz, Smoky Quartz with Aegerine

Kidneys, fortify: Grossular Garnet, Heulandite, Quartz

Kidneys, infection: Citrine, Yellow Zincite

Kidneys, regulating: Carnelian, Muscovite

Kidneys, stimulating: Rhodochrosite, Ruby

Kidneys, underactive: Fire Opal, Prehnite, Rhodochrosite, Ruby

Knees: Aragonite, Azurite, Blue Lace Agate, Cathedral Quartz, Charoite, Dinosaur Bone, Flint, Magnetite

– L –

Legs: Ametrine, Aquamarine, Bloodstone, Blue Tiger's Eye, Carnelian, Charoite, Garnet, Hawk's Eye, Jasper, Pietersite, Red Tiger's Eye, Ruby, Smoky Quartz, Tourmaline. *Chakra:* base, sacral, knees

Liver: Amber, Amethyst, Aquamarine, Azurite with Malachite, Beryl, Black Moonstone, Bloodstone, Blue Holly Agate, Brookite, Carnelian, Charoite, Chrysoprase, Cinnabar in Jasper, Citrine, Danburite, Eilat Stone,

Emerald, Empowerite, Epidote, Fluorite, Gaspeite, Gold Calcite, Golden Danburite, Guinea Fowl Jasper, Heulandite, Hiddenite, Hubnerite, Iolite, Labradorite, Lazulite, Lepidocrosite, Limonite, Orange River Quartz, Pietersite, Poppy Jasper, Red Amethyst, Red Jasper, Rhodonite, Rose Quartz, Ruby, Shungite, Tiger's Eye, Topaz, Tugtupite, Yellow Fluorite, Yellow Jasper, Yellow Labradorite. *Chakra:* dantien

Liver, blockages: Bastnasite, Fulgarite, Gaspeite, Holly Agate, Iolite, Orange Kyanite, Poppy Jasper, Red Jasper, Red Tourmaline, Rhodozite, Thunder Egg

Liver, blood flow: Mookaite Jasper

Liver, cleanse: Charoite, Crystal Cap Amethyst, Gaspeite, Iolite, Klinoptilolith, Peridot, Ruby

Liver, depletion: Holly Agate, Macedonian Opal, Tugtupite

Liver, stimulate: Amethyst, Azurite, Emerald, Poppy Jasper, Schalenblende, Silver Leaf Jasper, Tantalite, Thunder Egg, Tugtupite, Zircon

Lungs: Adamite, Amber, Amethyst, Ammolite, Andean Blue Opal, Atlantasite, Aventurine, Beryl, Blue Aragonite, Blue Quartz, Botswana Agate, Bustamite, Cacoxenite, Catlinite, Charoite, Chrysocolla, Diopside, Dioptase, Emerald, Fluorapatite, Fluorite, Graphic Smoky Quartz (Zebra Stone), Greenlandite, Hiddenite, Kambaba Jasper, Kunzite, Lapis Lazuli, Morganite, Peridot, Petalite, Petrified Wood, Pink Tourmaline, Prehnite, Prehnite with Epidote, Pyrite in Quartz, Quantum Quattro, Rhodochrosite, Rose Quartz, Sardonyx, Scheelite,

Scolecite, Serpentine, Serpentine in Obsidian, Smoky Amethyst, Sodalite, Sonora Sunrise, Stromatolite, Tremolite, Turquoise, Valentinite and Stibnite, Watermelon Tourmaline. *Chakra:* dantien, higher heart

Lungs, congested: Kambaba Jasper, Moss Agate, Quantum Quattro, Shungite, Stromatolite, Vanadinite

Lungs, difficulty in breathing: Anthrophyllite, Apophyllite, Chrysocolla, Green Siberian Quartz, Kambaba Jasper, Pietersite, Quantum Quattro, Riebekite with Sugilite and Bustamite, Stromatolite, Tremolite

Lungs, fluid in: Amber, Diamond, Hackmanite, Halite, Hanksite, Ocean Jasper, Scheelite, Smoky Amethyst, Yellow Sapphire, Zircon

Lymphatic, cleansing: Agate, Bastnasite, Chlorite Quartz, Crystal Cap Amethyst, Feather Pyrite, Ocean Jasper, Rose Quartz, Shungite, Sodalite, Sugilite, Yellow Apatite

Lymphatic, infections: Blue Lace Agate, Shungite

Lymphatic, stimulating: Bloodstone, Blue Chalcedony, Ocean Jasper, Oligocrase

Lymphatic, swellings: Agrellite, Anandalite™, Blue Euclase, Crystal Cap Amethyst, Jet

Lymphatic system: Agate, Anglesite, Bastnasite, Bloodstone, Blue Calcite, Blue Chalcedony, Chlorite Quartz, Eye of the Storm (Judy's Jasper), Graphic Smoky Quartz, Hackmanite, Lazulite, Moonstone, Moss Agate, Ocean Blue Jasper, Scheelite, Shungite, Tourmaline, Trigonic Quartz, Zebra Stone. *Chakra:* dantien, higher heart

Metabolic imbalances: Amazonite, Amechlorite, Azurite with Malachite and Chrysocolla, Blue Opal, Bornite, Champagne Aura Quartz, Chrysocolla, Diamond, Galaxyite, Garnet, Golden Azeztulite, Golden Danburite, Golden Herkimer, Hackmanite, Healer's Gold, Herkimer Diamond, Khutnohorite, Labradorite, Lemurian Jade, Mangano Vesuvianite, Peridot, Quantum Quattro, Que Sera, Shungite, Sonora Sunrise, Tantalite, Tanzine Aura Quartz, Tugtupite, Watermelon Tourmaline, Winchite. *Chakra:* dantien, third eye

Metabolic, stimulate processes: Apatite, Blue Tiger's Eye, Garnet, Hawk's Eye, Red Carnelian, Smoky Amethyst, Tugtupite. *Chakra:* brow and dantien

Metabolic syndrome: Amechlorite, Anandalite, Andara Glass, Galaxyite, Klinoptilolith, Quantum Quattro, Que Sera, Richterite, Scheelite, Shungite, Tanzine Aura Quartz, Winchite

Metabolic system: Amechlorite, Amethyst, Bloodstone, Carnelian, Champagne Aura Quartz, Hackmanite, Labradorite, Smoky Amethyst, Smoky Quartz with Aegerine, Sodalite, Tantalite, Winchite

Metabolism: Amazonite, Amechlorite, Ametrine, Bloodstone, Chrysoprase, Dendritic Agate, Fossilised Wood, Galaxyite, Garnet, Garnet in Pyroxene, Klinoptilolith, Labradorite, Quantum Quattro, Que Sera, Ruby, Serpentine, Shungite, Sodalite, Tourmaline, Tree Agate, Turquoise, Winchite

Metabolism, stimulate: Amethyst, Garnet, Pyrolusite,

Sodalite. *Chakra:* higher heart

Motor Dysfunction: Danburite, Kyanite, Sugilite

Muscle cramps: Apache Tear, Bastnasite, Cat's Eye Quartz, Celestite, Infinite Stone, Larimar, Magnesite, Magnetite (Lodestone), Orange Moss Agate, Quantum Quattro, Smithsonite Serpentine in Obsidian, Strontianite

Muscle disorders: Diopside, Kyanite, Peridot, Petalite, Rosophia

Muscle spasm: Amazonite, Apache Tear, Azurite with Malachite, Bornite, Chrysocolla, Diopside, Fuchsite, Magnetite (Lodestone), Malacholla, Petalite, Phlogopite, Pyrite in Magnesite, Red Tourmaline, Strontianite

Muscle tension: Basalt, Blue Aragonite, Blue Euclase, Champagne Aura Quartz

Muscle tension, release: Agate, Amazonite, Apatite, Aventurine, Azurite, Black Obsidian, Blue (Indicolite) Tourmaline, Blue Moonstone, Boji Stone, Brecciated Jasper, Celestite, Dravide (Brown) Tourmaline, Fuchsite, Hematite, Kundalini Quartz, Lapis Lazuli, Magnesite, Magnetite, Malachite, Obsidian, Pearl Spa Dolomite, Poppy Jasper, Selenite, Smoky Quartz, Stilbite, Tiger Iron, Tourmalinated Quartz

Muscle tissue: Aventurine, Danburite, Desert Rose, Khutnohorite, Magnetite (Lodestone), Phlogopite, Sonora Sunrise

Muscle tone: Fluorite, Peridot, Tourmaline

Muscles: Bismuth, Black Kyanite, Cat's Eye Quartz, Hematite, Jadeite, Nzuri Moyo, Petrified Wood, Phlogopite, Rhodonite, Scheelite, Titanite (Sphene)

Muscles, flexibility/pain: Aegerine, Blue Euclase, Cathedral Quartz, Eilat Stone, Flint, Rhodozite, Wind Fossil Agate

Muscles, strengthen: Aegerine, Apatite, Bismuth, Bustamite, Fluorite, Jadeite, Peridot, Tourmaline

Muscles, swelling: Anandalite™, Andean Blue Opal, Blue Euclase, Brochantite

Muscles, weak: Rhyolite, Tiger Iron

Muscular dystrophy: Rosophia, Scolecite and Natrolite

Musculoskeletal system inflexibility: Coprolite, Cumberlandite, Fuchsite, Jade, Kimberlite, Limonite, Magnesite, Quantum Quattro, Rosophia, Steatite, Stromatolite

– N –

Nerve endings: Guinea Fowl Jasper, Tinguaite

Nerve, pain relief: Blue Euclase, Flint, Nuummite, Rhodozite, Wind Fossil Agate

Nerves: Bronzite, Cat's Eye Quartz, Cryolite, Dalmatian Stone, Golden Coracalcite, Merlinite, Natrolite, Nuummite, Phlogopite, Scheelite, Scholecite, Smoky Amethyst, Stichtite, Tanzanite

Nerves, calming: Eudialyte, Jamesonite

Nerves, motor: Bustamite, Cat's Eye Quartz

Nerves, optic: see Alta major chakra page 107

Nerves, regenerating: Natrolite with Scolecite

Nerves, spinal: Tinguaite

Nerves, strengthen: Banded Agate, Drusy Quartz on Sphalerite, Mystic Topaz, Nuummite

Neural pathways: Golden Coracalcite, Larvikite, Merlinite, Mystic Merlinite, Natrolite, Scolecite, Stichtite, Phantom Calcite, Tree Agate

Neural transmission: Anglesite, Larvikite, Natrolite, Scolecite, Tremolite

Neurological tissue: Alexandrite, Golden Coracalcite, Natrolite, Phlogopite, Scolecite *and see Nerves above*

Neurotransmitters: Anglesite, Crystal Cap Amethyst, Golden Coracalcite, Kambaba Jasper, Khutnohorite, Ocean Blue Jasper, Phantom Calcite, Que Sera, Scolecite, Shungite, Sodalite, Stromatolite, Tremolite. *Chakra:* alta major (base of skull)

– P –

Pancreas: Amber, Astraline, Bloodstone, Blue Lace Agate, Brochantite, Bustamite, Carnelian, Charoite, Chinese Chromium Quartz, Chrysocolla, Citrine, Green Calcite, Hubnerite, Jasper, Leopardskin Jasper, Malachite, Maw Sit Sit, Moonstone, Pink Opal, Pink Tourmaline, Quantum Quattro, Red Tourmaline, Richterite, Schalenblende, Septarian, Serpentine in Obsidian, Shungite, Smoky Quartz, Tanzine Aura Quartz, Topaz, Tugtupite. *Chakra:* spleen, dantien

Pancreatic secretions: Astraline, Bustamite Muscovite, Malachite. *Chakra:* spleen, solar plexus, base *and see Blood sugar imbalances page 265*

Parathyroid: Blue Siberian Quartz, Cacoxenite, Champagne Aura Quartz, Chrysotile, Chrysotile in Serpentine, Cumberlandite, Kyanite, Leopardskin Jasper,

Malachite, Richterite, Tanzine Aura Quartz. *Chakra:* throat

Peripheral circulation: Aragonite, Dianite, Garnet in Quartz, Ouro Verde, Riebekite with Sugilite and Bustamite. *Chakra:* dantien

Pineal gland: Amethyst, Blue Moonstone, Champagne Aura Quartz, Fire and Ice Quartz, Fluorapatite, Gem Rhodonite, Moonstone, Opal, Petalite, Preseli Bluestone, Quartz, Richterite, Ruby, Tanzanite, Tanzine Aura Quartz, Tremolite Sodalite, Yellow Labradorite. *Chakra:* third eye

Pituitary gland: Apatite, Chalcopyrite, Champagne Aura Quartz, Charoite, Elbaite, Fire and Ice Quartz, Labradorite, Rhodonite, Sugilite, Tanzine Aura Quartz. *Chakra:* third eye

Prostate: Brochantite, Bustamite, Schalenblende. *Chakra:* base, sacral

Prostate, calming: Eudialyte, Jamesonite

Prostate, enlarged: Calcite Fairy Stone

Psoriasis: Conichalcite, Faden Quartz, Guinea Fowl Jasper, Snakeskin Agate, Wind Fossil Agate. *Bathe in essence or add to aqueous hydrating cream and rub in.*

– R –

Reproductive system: Beryllonite, Black Kyanite, Calcite Fairy Stone, Fire and Ice Quartz, Lepidocrosite, Menalite, Moonstone, Voegesite, Xenotine. *Chakra:* base, sacral, dantien

Reproductive system, fallopian tubes: Menalite,

Schalenblende. *Chakra:* sacral

Reproductive system, female: Black Moonstone, Fire and Ice Quartz, Menalite, Schalenblende, Tangerose. *Chakra:* sacral, base

Reproductive system, male: Calcite Fairy Stone, Schalenblende, Shiva Lingam

Reproductive system, ovaries: Menalite, Schalenblende

Reproductive system, testicles: Alexandrite, Schalenblende. *Chakra:* base

Respiratory problems: Cacoxenite, Kambaba Jasper, Riebekite with Sugilite and Bustamite, Smoky Amethyst, Stromatolite, Tremolite

Respiratory system: Blue Aragonite, Cacoxenite, Halite, Kambaba Jasper, Merlinite, Prophecy Stone, Pyrite in Quartz, Quantum Quattro, Richterite, Riebekite with Sugilite and Bustamite, Smoky Amethyst, Snakeskin Pyrite, Stromatolite, Tremolite. *Chakra:* dantien, higher heart

– S –

Skin: Agate, Amethyst, Aventurine, Azurite, Brown Jasper, Bustamite, Chohua Jasper, Eisenkiesel, Epidote, Ethiopian Opal, Faden Quartz, Galena *(caution: toxic)*, Green Jasper, Guinea Fowl Jasper, Halite, Hanksite, Honey Calcite, Kieseltuff, Klinoptilolith, Pearl Spa Dolomite, Phosphosiderite, Prehnite with Epidote, Riebekite with Sugilite and Bustamite, Rose Quartz, Snakeskin Agate, Stichtite, Sulphur *(caution: toxic)*, Titanite (Sphene), Topaz, Wind Fossil Agate. *Chakra:*

higher heart. *Or rub gently over site.*

Sympathetic nervous system: Cumberlandite, Golden Healer Quartz

T-cells: Bloodstone, Diaspore (Zultanite), Dioptase, Klinoptilolith, Quantum Quattro, Que Sera, Richterite, Rosophia, Shungite, Tangerine Sun Aura Quartz, Tangerose *and see Immune system page 291. Chakra:* higher heart

T-cells, encourage production: Diaspore, Golden Healer Quartz, Klinoptilolith, Shungite, Tangerose

Thymus: Amethyst, Andean Opal, Angelite, Aqua Aura, Aventurine, Bloodstone, Blue Halite, Blue or Green Tourmaline, Chrysotile, Citrine, Diaspore, Dioptase, Eilat Stone, Hiddenite, Indicolite Quartz, Jadeite, Klinoptilolith, Lapis Lazuli, Peridot, Prehnite with Epidote, Quantum Quattro, Quartz, Que Sera, Richterite, Rose Quartz, Septarian, Shaman Quartz, Stromatolite, Thompsonite, Tremolite. *Chakra:* higher heart

Thymus, underactive: Aqua Aura Quartz, Eilat Stone, Hiddenite, Lapis Lazuli, Peridot, Quantum Quattro, Que Sera, Smithsonite

Thyroid: Amber, Aqua Aura, Aquamarine, Azurite, Beryl, Blue Halite, Blue Tourmaline, Candle Quartz, Celestite, Champagne Aura Quartz, Citrine, Cryolite, Cumberlandite, Eilat Stone, Idocrase, Indicolite Quartz, Kyanite, Lapis Lazuli, Lavender Aura Quartz, Lazulite, Leopardskin Serpentine, Paraiba Tourmaline, Prehnite with Epidote, Quantum Quattro, Rhodonite, Richterite, Rutilated Quartz, Sapphire, Sodalite, Turquoise, Vanadinite. *Chakra:* throat

Thyroid, balance: Aquamarine, Cacoxenite, Richterite

Thyroid, deficiencies: Angelite, Blue Lace Agate, Citrine, Harlequin Quartz, Kyanite, Lapis Lazuli, Tanzine Aura Quartz

Thyroid, regulate: Lapis Lazuli, Rhodonite, Richterite, Tanzine Aura Quartz

Thyroid, stimulate: Rhodonite, Rutilated Quartz, Tanzine Aura Quartz. *Chakra:* throat

Stress and PTSD essences

Stress is estimated to be the underlying cause of around sixty per cent of illnesses and it is the core of PTSD. PTSD (post traumatic stress disorder) may occur from trauma in the recent or the far past, including ancestral sources, and may only make itself visible after many years of insidious operation. Physiological symptoms of stress include trembling, palpitations, and depression. The response is due to the body's 'fight or flight' survival mechanism. When a threat is perceived, or a memory triggered, the body gears up for violent muscular action. Adrenaline floods the system. Blood pressure rises, heart rate speeds up, and breathing accelerates. Pushing away or denying stress creates hyper-arousal. Stress becomes internalised, leading to pain, insomnia, anxiety, irregular heartbeat, high blood pressure, exhaustion, muscle tension, heart attack and strokes, or to overeating or malnutrition due to intestinal reactions.

Sounds familiar? Create an essence by choosing three or four crystals from the healing crystals for your most extreme symptoms. Your energy field will be highly sensitive so add a regulatory crystal from the list on page 52 or as indicated below and *begin by using one or two drops of the essence once a day, gradually increasing the amount up to seven drops three times a day.*

A-Z Directory

Choose 1–4 crystals from an entry when creating your essence.

– A –

Addictions: see page 187

Adrenal, balancing: Eye of the Storm, Fire Opal, Rose Quartz, Yellow Labradorite

Adrenal, calming: Cacoxenite, Eye of the Storm, Fire Opal, Green Calcite, Kyanite, Richterite, Rose Quartz, Yellow Labradorite

Adrenal overload: Aventurine, Eye of the Storm, Gaspeite, Grape Chalcedony, Jade, Lapis Lace, Nunderite, Picrolite, Richterite, Temple Calcite. *Chakra:* base, dantien (just below the navel), solar plexus (just above the navel). *Or rub over kidneys.*

Anger and tension, release: Alabaster, Blue Phantom Quartz, Chinese Red Quartz, Cinnabar in Jasper, Ethiopian Opal, Eye of the Storm, Greenlandite, Nzuri Moyo, Pearl Spa Dolomite, Phosphosiderite, Tugtupite, Ussingite. *Chakra:* base, dantien. *Or disperse essence around aura.*

Apathy: Carnelian, Chrysocolla, Garnet, Red Jasper, Triplite. *Chakra:* base and sacral, dantien

Arthritis: Azurite, Boji Stones, Chrysocolla, Malachite, Turquoise

Avoidance/denial: Apophyllite, Carnelian, Prehnite, Rhodochrosite. *Chakra:* heart

– B –

Blood pressure, equalize: Aventurine, Charoite, Eye of the Storm, Tourmaline. *Chakra:* heart, solar plexus

Blood pressure, high: Amethyst, Bloodstone, Blue Chalcedony, Charoite, Chrysocolla, Chrysoprase, Dioptase, Emerald, Eye of the Storm (Green), Jade, Kyanite, Labradorite, Lapis Lazuli, Malachite, Rhodochrosite, Sodalite. *Chakra:* heart

Blood pressure, low: Carnelian, Eye of the Storm (orange/brown), Red Calcite, Rhodochrosite, Ruby, Sodalite, Tourmaline. *Chakra:* heart

– C –

Chronic anxiety: Amethyst, Chrysocolla, Eye of the Storm, Grape Chalcedony, Kunzite, Lapis Lace, Prairie Tanzanite. *Chakra:* heart

Communication, higher: Carnelian, Chrysoberyl, Datolite, Diamond, Fluorite, Goethite, Green Tourmaline, Hematite, Herderite, Jade, Lapis Lazuli, Magnetite, Malachite, Obsidian, Red Jasper, Ruby, Schalenblende. *Chakra:* third eye

Communication problems: Blue Lace Agate, Chrysocolla, Lapis Lace, Lapis Lazuli, Sodalite, Turquoise. *Chakra:* heart

Compulsive thoughts: Auralite 23, Banded Agate, Blue Kyanite, Fluorite, Freedom Stone, Grape Chalcedony, Herkimer Diamond, Rhomboid Selenite. *Chakra:* third eye, past life

Confusion, disperse: Amethyst, Azurite, Bloodstone, Blue Scapolite, Carnelian, Celestial Quartz, Charoite, Crystal Cap Amethyst, Elestial Quartz, Fluorite, Gabbro, Hematoid Calcite, Howlite, Kakortokite, Lapis Lazuli, Lepidocrosite, Limonite, Magnetite, Opal, Owyhee Blue Opal, Paraiba Tourmaline, Pietersite, Quartz, Rhodochrosite, Sapphire, Selenite, Sodalite. *Chakra:* between third eye and soma

Courage needed: Carnelian, Red Jasper. *Chakra:* base and sacred

– D –

Depression: Ajo Blue Calcite, Amber, Amethyst, Ametrine, Apatite, Apophyllite, Botswana Agate, Carnelian, Chrysoprase, Citrine, Clinohumite, Dianite, Eisenkiesel, Eudialyte, Flint, Garnet, Golden Healer, Green Ridge Quartz, Hematite, Idocrase, Jade, Jet, Kunzite, Lapis Lazuli, Lepidolite, Lithium Quartz, Macedonian Opal, Maw Sit Sit, Montebrasite, Moss Agate, Orange Kyanite, Pink Sunstone, Porphyrite (Chinese Letter Stone), Purple Tourmaline, Rainbow Geothite, Rutilated Quartz, Siberian Quartz, Sillimanite, Smoky Quartz, Spessarite Garnet, Spiders Web Obsidian, Spinel, Staurolite, Sunstone, Tiger's Eye, Tugtupite, Turquoise. *Chakra:* solar plexus

Disconnection from Earth: Flint, Granite, Hematite, Lemurian Jade, Libyan Gold Tektite, Preseli Bluestone, Quartz, Smoky Elestial Quartz, Strontianite, Tektite *and see Grounding. Chakra:* dantien, soma, earth star, Gaia gateway

Dis-ease due to stress: Amechlorite, Basalt, Bird's Eye Jasper, Black Moonstone, Eye of the Storm, Galaxyite, Lemurian Gold Opal, Macedonian Opal, Marble, Orgonite, Richterite, Riebekite with Sugilite and Bustamite, Shungite, Tektite, Tugtupite *and see Stress page 293*

Dizziness: Aragonite, Candle Quartz, Cathedral Quartz, Dioptase, Eye of the Storm, Flint, Golden Healer Quartz, Hematite, Lapis Lazuli, Mohawkite, Poppy Jasper, Quartz, Richterite, White Sapphire. *Chakra:* dantien, crown

– F –

Flashbacks/Intrusive memories: Ancestralite, Auralite 23, Banded Agate, Brandenberg Amethyst, Datolite, Grape Chalcedony, Lepidolite, Nuummite. *Chakra:* third eye and past life

Frustration: Blue Lace Agate, Grape Chalcedony, Lapis Lace, Prairie Tanzanite, Red Jasper, Rhodochrosite, Rhodonite, Rose Quartz. *Chakra:* base, sacral, heart

– G –

Guilt, survivor: Aquamarine, Chrysocolla, Garnet, Mangano Calcite, Rose Quartz. *Chakra:* solar plexus

– H –

Helplessness: Black Tourmaline, Carnelian, Garnet, Lapis Lazuli. *Chakra:* dantien, base and sacral

Hopelessness: Amethyst, Anandalite, Aquamarine, Lepidolite. *Chakra:* heart

Hyper-vigilance: Anandalite, Auralite 23, Flint, Grape Chalcedony, Labradorite, Lepidolite, Petrified Wood, Selenite, Tanzurine. *Chakra:* heart, third eye

– I –

Immune system support: Bloodstone, Fluorite, Green Aventurine, Green Calcite, Quantum Quattro, Que Sera (Llanoite), Tanzurine. *Chakra:* higher heart

Insomnia: Amethyst, Auralite 23, Bloodstone, Jade, Labradorite, Lepidolite, Sodalite. Drop essence on to pillow.

Irritability: Garnet, Grape Chalcedony, Lepidolite, Rhodonite, Rose Quartz

Isolation: Garnet, Grape Chalcedony, Labradorite, Red Jasper, Septarian, Spirit Quartz. *Chakra:* heart seed, base, sacral and navel

– L –

Lack of feelings: Dioptase, Grape Chalcedony, Rose Quartz, Smoky Quartz, Topaz. *Chakra:* solar plexus

Loss of motivation: Carnelian, Chrysocolla, Red Jasper, Red Tiger's Eye, Ruby. *Chakra:* dantien, base, sacral

Low self-esteem: Carnelian, Cinnabar (*caution: toxic*), Citrine, Prehnite, Triplite

– M –

Mistrust: Amethyst, Anandalite, Grape Chalcedony, Prairie

Tanzanite, Rosophia, Topaz, Turquoise. *Chakra:* heart

– N –

Negative self-image: Carnelian, Citrine, Golden Calcite, Rose Quartz, Sodalite. *Chakra:* heart

Nightmares: Amethyst, Auralite 23, Bloodstone, Charoite, Jade, Lepidolite, Rose Quartz, Sodalite. Drop essence on to pillow.

– P –

Palpitations/Tachycardia: Amber, Brandenberg Amethyst, Chrysoprase, Emerald, Garnet, Jade, Morganite, Preseli Bluestone (*caution: use with regulatory crystal, see page 52*), Rhodochrosite, Rose Quartz, Ruby, Tiger's Eye, Tugtupite. *Chakra:* heart seed, higher heart, heart, earth star, Gaia gateway, knee

Panic attack: Amazonite, Amethyst, Ancestralite, Aquamarine, Aventurine, Blue-green Smithsonite, Brandenberg Amethyst, Celtic Chevron Quartz, Charoite, Cradle of Humankind, Dumortierite, Eye of the Storm, Girasol, Grape Chalcedony, Green Phantom Quartz, Green Tourmaline, Kunzite, Lakelandite, Larimar, Morganite, Prairie Tanzanite, Rhodonite, Rose Quartz, Serpentine in Obsidian, Tremolite, Turquoise. *Chakra:* heart, higher heart, solar plexus. Spray around aura.

Physical pain: Azurite, Cathedral Quartz, Lapis Lazuli, Smoky Quartz, Sugilite. *Chakra:* heart, *or rub over site*

Poor concentration: Banded Agate, Brandenberg Amethyst, Fluorite, Lepidolite, Sodalite. *Chakra:* third eye

Poor judgement: Brandenberg Amethyst, Fluorite,

Sodalite. *Chakra:* third eye

– R –

Rage: Amethyst, Eye of the Storm, Hematite, Prairie Tanzanite, Rhodonite, Rose Quartz, Selenite

Regulatory crystals: Eye of the Storm, Herkimer Diamond, Quartz *and see page 52*

– S –

Short-term memory loss: Brandenberg Amethyst, Carnelian, Fluorite, Sodalite. *Chakra:* third eye

Soul loss from extreme trauma: Black Tourmaline, Flint, Hematite, Nuummite, Selenite. *Chakra:* heart, soma

Spleen: Aegerine, Amber, Apple Aura Quartz, Aquamarine, Aventurine, Azurite, Black Moonstone, Bloodstone, Blue Quartz, Brochantite, Bustamite, Chalcedony, Cinnabar in Jasper, Citrine, Fluorite, Gaspeite, Green Obsidian, Guinea Fowl Jasper, Jade, Marcasite, Mookaite Jasper, Nunderite, Orange River Quartz, Peridot, Red Obsidian, Red Tourmaline, Ruby, Septarian, Sunstone, Yellow Labradorite, Wulfenite, Zircon. *Chakra:* spleen

Spleen, blood flow: Mookaite Jasper

Spleen deterioration: Mookaite Jasper, Prasiolite

Spleen, detoxifying: Amechlorite, Banded Agate, Chlorite Quartz, Eye of the Storm, Jamesonite, Larvikite, Pyrite in Magnesite, Rainbow Covellite, Richterite, Seraphinite, Shungite, Smoky Quartz with Aegerine

Spleen protection: Aventurine, Gaspeite, Green Aventurine, Jade, Nunderite, Tugtupite

Stress: Amethyst, Auralite 23, Basalt, Bird's Eye Jasper, Bustamite, Charoite, Eudialyte, Eye of the Storm, Grape Chalcedony, Larvikite, Marble, Merlinite, Prairie Tanzanite, Rhodochrosite, Richterite, Riebekite with Sugilite and Bustamite, Rose Quartz, Shungite, Tugtupite
Survivor guilt: Anandalite, Chrysocolla, Cradle of Life (Humanity), Flint, Freedom Stone, Isua, Jade, Nuummite, Rose Quartz, Selenite. *Chakra:* heart and solar plexus

– T –

Trembling/twitching: Aragonite, Magnesite, Magnetite, Rhodozite

– U –

Ulcers: Ametrine, Calcite, Chrysocolla, Fluorite, Green Aventurine, Sunstone

Useful adult essences

When family members live together, their energies are so involved with each other that we have found it more effective to treat all members of the family, and that this really gets results.
– Petaltone Essences

In addition to the other purpose-made essences listed in the book, you may find these essences useful for emergency first aid and other situations.

Choose 1–4 crystals from an entry when creating your essence.

A-Z Directory

– A –

Anaphylactic shock: Ouro Verde, Richterite, Tantalite. *Chakra:* dantien, heart, higher heart

Antibacterial and antiviral (coughs, colds, flu): Amber, Anhydrite, Bloodstone, Blue Euclase, Blue Tourmaline (Indicolite), Cathedral Quartz, Golden Healer Quartz, Green Calcite, Honey Opal, Iolite, Malachite, Owyhee Blue Opal, Proustite, Quantum Quattro, Que Sera, Shungite, Sulphur, Sulphur in Quartz, Trummer Jasper, Wonder Stone. *Chakra:* higher heart. Bathe in crystal essence, drink Shungite activated water.

– B –

Breathlessness: Amber, Amethyst, Apophyllite, Black Onyx, Jet, Kambaba Jasper, Magnetite (Lodestone), Morganite, Moss Agate, Quantum Quattro, Que Sera, Stromatolite, Vanadinite. *Chakra:* higher heart, solar plexus, throat

Bronchitis: Amber, Black Onyx, Iron Pyrite, Jet, Kambaba Jasper, Pyrolusite, Rutilated Quartz, Shungite, Stromatolite

Burns: Amphibole, Hemimorphite, Indicolite, Klinoptilolith, Lilac Quartz, Rose Quartz

– C –

Cancer: Eilat Stone, Fluorapatite, Gabbro, Klinoptilolith, Malacolla, Rhodozite, Shungite water, Sonora Sunrise *and*

see EMF page 231

support during: Amethyst Spirit Quartz, Bixbite, Black Diopside, Brandenberg Amethyst, Cassiterite, Cathedral Quartz, Cobolto Calcite, Dendritic Chalcedony, Epidote, Eye of the Storm, Green Ridge Quartz, Hemimorphite, Icicle Calcite, Lemurian Jade, Paraiba Tourmaline, Quantum Quattro, Reinerite, Rhodozite, Sonora Sunrise, Tremolite, Winchite

Carpal tunnel syndrome: Eye of the Storm, Fuchsite, Magnetite (Lodestone), Spider Web Jasper. *Rub over site.*

Centring essence: Bloodstone, Calcite, Celestobarite, Coral", Eye of the Storm, Flint, Fossilised Wood, Garnet, Hematite, Kunzite, Obsidian, Onyx, Peanut Wood, Quartz, Red Jasper, Ruby, Sardonyx, Tourmalinated Quartz. *Chakra:* Gaia gateway, earth star, base, dantien

Conception: Menalite, Moonstone, Rose Quartz

– D –

'Defragging' crystals: Anandalite, Ancestralite, Brandenberg Amethyst, Celtic Quartz, Cradle of Life (Humanity), Golden Lemurian Seed, Iolite-and-Sunstone, Lapis Lace, Rainbow Lattice Sunstone, Rainbow Mayanite, Sea Foam Flint, Strawberry Lemurian Seed

Diarrhoea: Green Tourmaline, Lapis Lazuli, Malachite, Pearl, Quartz, Serpentine

– F –

First aid: Eye of the Storm, Garnet in Quartz, Quantum Quattro, Que Sera, Richterite, Tangerose, Tantalite.

Chakra: dantien, higher heart. *Disperse around aura.*

Food poisoning: Amber, Shungite water

Forgetfulness: Chlorite Quartz, Emerald, Eye of the Storm, Golden Healer Quartz, Moss Agate, Poppy Jasper, Rhodonite, Sodalite, Tourmaline, Unakite. *Chakra:* brow

– H –

Headache: Amber, Amblygonite, Blue Sapphire, Bustamite, Cathedral Quartz, Champagne Aura Quartz, Dioptase, Dumortierite, Galena (*caution: toxic*), Greenlandite, Hematite, Jet, Lapis Lazuli, Magnesite, Pyrite in Magnesite, Quantum Quattro, Rhodozite, Rose Quartz, Smoky Quartz, Sugilite, Turquoise. *Chakra:* third eye

Headache arising from neck tension: Cathedral Quartz, Magnetite (Lodestone), Quantum Quattro. On base of skull.

Headache, blocked alta major chakra: Blue Moonstone, Garnet in Pyroxene, Herderite, Orange Kyanite, Rhomboid Selenite, Riebekite with Sugilite and Bustamite, *and see Alta major chakra page 107*

Hearing loss: Alabandite, Ammolite, Budd Stone (African Jade), Kambaba Jasper, Leopardskin Serpentine, Peanut Wood, Smoky Amethyst, Snakeskin Agate, Stromatolite. *Chakra:* past life

Hot flushes/flashes and night sweats: Aquamarine, Blue Lace Agate, Blue Tourmaline, Calcite, Citrine, Dumortierite in Quartz, Fire Agate, Gaia Flint, Garnet, Green Aventurine, Indicolite Quartz, Jade, Kundalini

Quartz, Lapis Lace, Lapis Lazuli, Larimar, Lepidolite, Lithium, Menalite, Moonstone, Rhodolite Garnet, Rose Quartz, Ruby, Shiva Lingam, Smoky Quartz, Sunstone-and-Iolite, Tanzine Aura Quartz (indium alchemicalised, not dyed), Triplite in matrix. *Chakra:* sacral. *Disperse essence around aura and pillow. Consider treating stuck kundalini* (see *Crystal Prescriptions 4*).

– I –

Influenza: Fluorite, Moss Agate, Quantum Quattro, Que Sera, Shungite. *Chakra:* higher heart

– J –

Jetlag: Preseli Bluestone, Shungite

– M –

Migraine: Amethyst, Aventurine, Azurite, Cathedral Quartz, Dioptase, Iolite, Jet, Lapis Lazuli, Magnesite, Pearl, Rhodochrosite, Rose Quartz, Sodalite, Sugilite, Topaz. *Chakra:* brow, crown, past life

– P –

Pain relief: Amber, Amethyst, Aragonite, Boji Stones, Cathedral Quartz, Celestite, Dendritic Agate, Fluorite, Hematite, Infinite Stone, Lapis Lazuli, Larimar, Magnetite (Lodestone), Mahogany Obsidian, Malachite, Quartz, Rose Quartz, Seraphinite, Smoky Quartz, Sugilite, Tourmaline

PMS: Bastnasite, Beryllonite, Blue Euclase, Labradorite,

Lodalite, Menalite, Moonstone, Nephrite Jade, Orange Kyanite, Quantum Quattro, Rhodozite, Serpentine in Obsidian, Smoky Quartz, Yellow or Picture Jasper. *Chakra:* sacral

Preservatives: Brandy, Cider Vinegar, Citricidal, Glycerol, Shungite, Vodka, White Rum. Essential oils: frankincense, lavender, myrrh, sage.

Psoriasis: Conichalcite, Faden Quartz, Guinea Fowl Jasper, Snakeskin Agate, Wind Fossil Agate. *Bathe in essence or add to aqueous hydrating cream and rub in.*

– R –

Regulatory crystals: Aragonite, Black Kyanite, Calcite, Charoite, Chromium Quartz, Fluorite, Green Kyanite, Halite, Isua, Kiwi Stone (Sesame Jasper), Ocean Jasper, Prairie Tanzanite, Quartz, Rose Quartz, Selenite, Serpentine, Shungite, Smoky Quartz, Tanzurine (Cherry and Emerald Quartz)

Road/transport rage, ameliorate: Amethyst, Chrysocolla, Garnet, Rhodonite, Rose Quartz, Shungite

– S –

Seasonal affective disorder: Sunshine Aura Quartz, Sunstone, Topaz, Triplite. *Chakra:* sacral, solar plexus, higher heart. *Rub on wrists several times a day.*

Senile dementia: Anthrophyllite, Blue Moonstone, Brandenberg Amethyst, Chalcedony, Fluorite, Rose Quartz, Stichtite and Serpentine. *Chakra:* third eye, alta major (base of skull). *Bathe or sip several times a day.*

Senior moments: Barite, Blue or Black Moonstone, Hematoid Calcite, Herderite, Marcasite, Vivianite. *Chakra:* third eye. *Rub at base of skull.*

Sensitivity to lightning: Agate, Amethyst, Fulgarite, Lightning Strike Quartz, Pietersite, Shungite. *Chakra:* crown

Shield: Black Tourmaline, Healer's Gold, Master Shamanite, Nuummite, Polychrome Jasper, Pyrite, Shieldite, Shungite, Smoky Quartz, Tantalite. *Chakra:* higher heart

Sleep: see Insomnia page 291

Spasms: Amazonite, Aragonite, Azurite, Carnelian, Electric-blue Obsidian, Magnesite, Ruby

Stress: see Stress and PTSD

– T –

Tachycardia: see Stress and PTSD

Tie-cutting: Charoite, Flint, Green Aventurine, Rainbow Mayanite, Rainbow Obsidian. *Chakra:* spleen and solar plexus

Tiredness, chronic: Amethyst, Bismuth, Carnelian, Chlorite Quartz, Cinnabar in Jasper, Eudialyte, Eye of the Storm, Fire Agate, Fire Obsidian, Golden Healer Quartz, Hematite, Iron Pyrite, Poppy Jasper, Purpurite, Quantum Quattro, Que Sera, Red Jasper, Rose Quartz, Ruby, Ruby in Fuchsite, Tiger Iron, Triplite, *and see Chronic fatigue page 267. Chakra:* base, dantien

Toxins, disperse: Actinolite, Aegerine, Ametrine, Banded Agate, Barite, Blue Quartz, Celestite, Celestobarite,

Champagne Aura Quartz, Chinese Chromium Quartz, Chlorite Quartz, Chrysanthemum Stone, Conichalcite, Covellite, Danburite with Chlorite, Eilat Stone, Epidote, Eye of the Storm, Fairy Quartz, Fiskenaesset Ruby, Golden Danburite, Halite, Hanksite, Hubnerite, Iolite, Leopardskin Serpentine, Morion, Ocean Jasper, Orgonite, Pearl Spa Dolomite, Poppy Jasper, Pumice, Pyrite in Quartz, Quantum Quattro, Seraphinite, Serpentine, Shieldite, Smoky Elestial Quartz, Smoky Herkimer, Snakeskin Pyrite, Sodalite, Spirit Quartz, Yellow Apatite. *Chakra:* base, earth star, dantien, spleen, solar plexus. *And see Detoxification page 230.*

Travel support: Orgonite, Preseli Bluestone, Shieldite, Shungite, Smoky Quartz

– U –

Ungroundedness: Aztee, Basalt, Celestobarite, Chlorite Quartz, Dragon Stone, Empowerite, Flint, Granite, Graphic Smoky Quartz (Zebra Stone), Hematite, Kambaba Jasper, Mohawkite, Peanut Wood, Polychrome Jasper, Proustite, Serpentine in Obsidian, Shell Jasper, Smoky Elestial Quartz, Steatite, Stromatolite. *Chakra:* earth star, base, dantien. *Or rub behind knees.*

– V –

Vertigo: Celestobarite, Dogs Tooth Calcite, Fairy Quartz, Zircon (*rub on back of neck*)

– W –

Weather sensitivity: Apricot Quartz, Avalonite, Chlorite Quartz, Golden Healer Quartz, Golden Pietersite, Khutnohorite, Quantum Quattro, Que Sera, Poppy Jasper, Shell Jasper, Shungite, Sillimanite, Silver Leaf Jasper, Trummer Jasper, Wonder Stone. *Chakra:* third eye
Winter blues: Citrine, Quartz, Selenite, Sunstone, Sunstone-and-Iolite. *Chakra:* higher heart

»Always use ethically sourced Coral.

Young people's essences

Crystal essences are particularly helpful for children and young people as they work gently and intelligently. Brains are particularly 'plastic' at this stage of life and can be repatterned to work more effectively through adjusting the etheric blueprint so that the effect filters into the physical. Regulatory crystals (see page 52) can be added to an essence to ensure that the essence radiates exactly the right amount of energy and at the rate that is appropriate for the recipient. Children's essences should be dispersed around the aura, added to bathwater or gently rubbed over an appropriate chakra or organ.

Choose 1–4 crystals from an entry when creating your essence. Add regulatory crystals where appropriate.

A-Z Directory

– A –

Allergies: Aquamarine, Aventurine, Carnelian, Fluorite, Garnet, Red Jasper, Snakeskin Agate. *Chakra:* palm, sacral, third eye

Anorexia: Azotic Topaz, Mystic Topaz, Orange Kyanite, Picasso Jasper, Tugtupite. *Chakra:* earth star, base, heart

Antisocial behaviour: Atlantasite, Blizzard Stone, Stichtite. *Disperse around aura and environment.*

Asthma: Amber, Amethyst, Ametrine, Apophyllite, Chrysoberyl, Dark-blue Sapphire, Iron Pyrite, Magnetite (Lodestone), Malachite, Morganite, Rhodochrosite, Rose Quartz, Tiger's Eye, Topaz, Vanadinite. *Chakra:* solar plexus, higher heart

ADHD (Attention deficit hyperactivity disorder): Amblygonite, Brandenberg Amethyst, Cumberlandite, Kunzite, Lepidocrosite, Lithium Quartz, Rutilated Quartz, Stichtite, Tantalite, Tanzine Aura Quartz. *Chakra:* dantien. *Disperse around aura.*

Attitude, to change: Amethyst Spirit Quartz, Axinite, Dream Quartz, Drusy Danburite, Eclipse Stone, Fluorapatite, Heulandite, Lilac Crackle Quartz, Luxullianite, Purpurite, Satyaloka Quartz, Smoky Citrine, Stichtite, Wavellite

Autism spectrum: Black Amber, Black Moonstone, Cerussite (*caution: toxic*), Charoite, Flint, Fluorite, Gaia's Blood (Red) Flint, Hematite, Moldavite, Sugilite *and see Protection (page 236) and Grounding (page 226). Chakra:*

earth, base, solar plexus. *Sequence:* stellar gateway and Gaia gateway; soul star and earth star; crown and base; third eye and dantien. *Or apply essences to soles of feet.*

– B –

Body dysmorphia: Dianite

Bulimia: Dianite, Orange Kyanite, Picasso Jasper. *Chakra:* solar plexus

Bullying: Carnelian, Cat's Eye Quartz, Red Jasper, Shiva Lingam. *Chakra:* dantien. *Or disperse around aura. And see Authority figures and Autonomy, page 249.*

– C –

Chicken pox/herpes: Dalmatian Stone, Fluorite, Guinea Fowl Jasper, Quantum Quattro, Que Sera, Shungite, Silver Agate, Smoky Quartz, Tanzurine (Cherry and Emerald Quartz)

Childhood, enjoyment: Crackle Quartz, Dalmatian Stone, Goldstone, Kiwi Jasper, Smoky Quartz, Sugilite, White-Sodalite

Confidence: Carnelian, Cat's Eye Quartz, Empowerite, Strontianite, Tremolite. *Disperse around aura.*

Crystal children: Anandalite, Aura Quartzes, bicoloured stones, Flint, Hematite, Iolite. All the new high-vibration Quartz crystals, *plus Protection (see page 236) and Grounding stones (see page 226). Disperse essence around the aura.*

– D –

Down's syndrome: Amazez, Amethyst Aura Quartz, Ametrine, Anandalite, Auralite 24, Blue or Milky Way Flint, Champagne Aura Quartz, Chrysoprase, Danburite, Fluorite, Garnet, Labradorite, Morganite, Rhodochrosite, Rhodonite, Rose Quartz, Selenite, Tiger Iron. *Chakra:* crown. *Chakra sequence:* base and crown; earth star and soul star; Gaia gateway and stellar gateway. *Disperse essence around the head.*

Dyslexia: Black Moonstone, Scapolite, Sodalite, Sugilite. *Chakra:* third eye, alta major

Dyspraxia: Black Moonstone, Red Muscovite, Smoky Quartz, Sodalite, Sugilite. *Chakra:* third eye, alta major

– E –

Eating disorders: Sichuan Quartz, Sugilite, Tibetan Black Spot Quartz *and see appropriate entries in Addictions*

Eczema: Agate, Amethyst, Green Aventurine, Ocean Jasper, Sapphire, Selenite, Snakeskin Agate. *Bathe with alcohol-free crystal essence.*

Examinations/studying: Calcite, Chalcedony, Fluorite, Green Aventurine, Muscovite, Quartz, Sodalite, Turquoise. *Disperse around head.*

– H –

Hyperactivity: Black Moonstone, Cerussite (*caution: toxic*), Cumberlandite, Dianite, Fiskenaesset Ruby, Garnet, Grape Chalcedony, Green Tourmaline, Lepidocrosite, Montebrasite, Moonstone, Pearl Spa

Dolomite, Prairie Tanzanite, Sugilite, Yellow Scapolite and *see Grounding crystals page 226. Chakra:* earth star, base, dantien *and see ADHD page 305*

Hypersensitivity: Dumortierite, Proustite *and see Delicate/sensitive people, page 319*

– I –

Indigo children: Amethyst, Angelite, Aquamarine, Atlantasite, Black Moonstone, Bloodstone, Charoite, Flint, Garnet, Hematite, Iolite, Labradorite, Rhomboid Selenite, Ruby, Selenite, Smoky Quartz, Spectrolite, Tanzanite, Tanzine Aura Quartz, White Labradorite. *Chakra:* stellar gateway and Gaia gateway, soul star and earth star; base and sacral, *and see Protection page 236 and Grounding stones page 226*

Itching: Agate, Aquamarine, Rose Quartz, Selenite, Snakeskin Agate. *Bathe affected parts with non-alcohol-preserved essence.*

– L –

Learning difficulties: Annabergite, Black Moonstone, Sugilite. *Chakra:* third eye, crown, alta major

Linguistic capability: Annabergite, Calligraphy Stone, Chinese Writing Stone, Dumortierite, Novaculite. *Chakra:* throat, third eye, soma

– M –

Measles: Dalmatian Stone, Leopardskin Jasper, Rosasite, Topaz, Turquoise

Mumps: Aquamarine, Topaz

M.E. (Myalgic encephalomyelitis): Ametrine, Bismuth, Chinese Red Quartz, Chrysolite in Serpentine, Eye of the Storm, Petrified Wood, Quantum Quattro, Que Sera, Ruby, Shungite, Tourmaline. *Chakra:* dantien, higher heart

– N –

Nausea: Brown Agate, Dioptase, Emerald, Fuchsite, Green Calcite, Green Jasper, Red Aventurine, Sapphire. *Chakra:* solar plexus

New friends: Chrysoprase, Jade, Spider Web Jasper

Nightmares/night terrors: Dalmatian Stone, Fairy Quartz, Smoky Quartz, Sodalite, Spirit Quartz, Tourmaline, Tremolite. *Chakra:* third eye. *And see pages 292.*

– S –

Speech impediments/stammering: Black Moonstone, Blue Crackle Quartz, Blue Euclase, Blue Lace Agate, Fluorite, Sodalite, Spiders Web Obsidian, Sugilite. *Chakra:* third eye, throat

Star children: Calcite Fairy Stone, Empowerite, Fairy Quartz, Glaucophane, Star Hollandite, Starseed Quartz. *Chakra:* higher crown

Startle response: Blue Moonstone, Brandenberg Amethyst, Sodalite. *Rub on back of neck.*

– T –

Teething pain: Blue Euclase, Cathedral Quartz, Quantum

Quattro, Rhodozite

Temper tantrums: Eye of the Storm, Grape Chalcedony, Neptunite, Pearl Spa Dolomite, Prairie Tanzanite, Rose Quartz, Selenite. *Chakra:* base, dantien

Temperature, regulate: Crackled Fire Agate, Dinosaur Bone, Madagascan Green Opal, Nuummite, Pyrite in Magnesite. *Rub beside left ear.*

Toothache: Cathedral Quartz, Quantum Quattro, Shungite

Tourette's syndrome: Eye of the Storm, Fenster Quartz

Tranquillizer: Amblygonite, Blue Quartz, Candle Quartz, Eye of the Storm, Grape Chalcedony, Leopardskin Jasper, Poppy Jasper, Pounamou Jade, Prairie Tanzanite, Quantum Quattro, Strawberry Quartz, Vera Cruz Amethyst. *Chakra:* higher heart

– W –

Warts: Flint, Hemimorphite, Snakeskin Agate

Contraindications

Please note: The following crystals may contain trace amounts of toxic minerals and should be used in tumbled form wherever possible. Do not inhale dust. Create essences by the indirect method and wash hands after handling. This information is given so that you can make up your own mind about their use. The list is updated regularly on my website: www.judyhall.co.uk.

A-Z Directory

A

Actinolite: asbestos
Adamite: arsenic and copper
Ajoite: aluminium and copper
Alexandrite: aluminium
Almandine Garnet: aluminium
Amazonite: copper
Amblygonite: aluminium
Andaluscite: aluminium
Angelite: calcium sulphate, lead
Anhydrate: calcium sulphate, lead
Aquamarine: aluminium
Aragonite: toxic when burnt
Arsenopyrite: iron arsenic sulphide
Atacamite: copper
Auricalcite: zinc and copper
Aventurine: aluminium
Axinite: aluminium, iron
Azurite: copper

B

Bastnasite: toxic in water
Beryl: aluminium
Beryllium: beryllium
Biotite: iron
Bixbite: aluminium
Black Tourmaline: aluminium

Boji Stones: pyrite, marcasite, sulphur
Bornite: copper iron sulphide
Brazilianite: aluminium
Bronchantite: copper hydrated sulphate
Bronzite: iron
Bumble Bee Jasper: sulphur, realgar and orpiment

C
Cassiterite: tin oxide
Cavansite: calcium vanadium silicate
Celestite: strontium sulphate
Celtic Quartz: possibility of lead
Cerrusite: lead carbonate
Chalchantite: copper, sulphur
Chalcopyrite: copper and sulphur
Chrome Diopside: copper
Chryolite: aluminium sodium fluoride
Chrysoberyl: aluminium
Chrysocolla: copper
Chrysotile: asbestos
Cinnabar: mercury sulphide
Conichalcite: copper, arsenic
Copper: unbound copper
Covellite: copper sulphide
Crocoite: chromium
Cuprite: copper

D
Dalmatian Jasper: aluminium

Dioptase: copper cyclosilicate
Dumortierite: aluminium

E
Eilat Stone: copper
Emerald: aluminium
Epidote: aluminium
Eudialyte: mildly radioactive

F
Feldspar: aluminium
Fluorite: fluoride

G
Galena: lead
Garnierite (Falcondoite/Genthite): nickel
Gem Silica: copper
Germanium: unbound germanium
Golden Celtic Quartz: possibility of lead
Goshenite: aluminium

H
Heliodor: aluminium
Hematite: iron
Hessonite Garnet: aluminium
Hiddenite: aluminium

I
Idocrase: aluminium

Iolite: aluminium

J
Jadeite: aluminium, iron
Jamesonite: antimony (lead)

K
Kinoite: hydrated calcium copper silicate
Klinoptilolith: volcanic ash
Kunzite: aluminium
Kyanite: aluminium

L
Labradorite: aluminium
Lapis Lazuli: sulphur, pyrite
Lazulite: aluminium
Lazurite: aluminium, sulphur
Lemon Chrysoprase: nickel Magnesite
Lepidolite: aluminium

M
Magnetite: iron
Malachite: copper
Malacholla: copper
Marcasite: may convert to sulphuric acid powder
Messina Quartz: copper
Mica: aluminium
Mohawkite: copper, arsenic
Moldavite: aluminium oxide

Molybdenum: lead
Moonstone: aluminium
Moqui Balls: iron
Morganite: aluminium
Muscovite: aluminium

O
Orpiment: arsenic. *Highly toxic.*
Orthoclase: aluminium

P
Pargasite: aluminium
Peacock Ore: copper and sulphur
Pietersite: asbestos
Plancheite: hydrated copper silicate
Prehnite: aluminium
Psilomelane: barium
Pyrite: iron and sulphur
Pyromorphite: lead

Q
Quantum Quattro: copper
Que Sera: copper

R
Realgar: arsenic. *Highly toxic.*
Realgar and Orpiment: arsenic, lead. *Highly toxic.*
Renierite: germanium
Rhodolite Garnet: aluminium

Rubellite: aluminium
Ruby: aluminium

S

Sapphire: aluminium
Scapolite: aluminium
Schorl: aluminium
Serpentine: asbestos
Shattuckite: copper
Shungite (Elite or Noble): may contain pyrite
Smithsonite: zinc, copper (green)
Sodalite: aluminium
Spessartine Garnet: aluminium
Sphalerite: zinc sulphide
Spinel: aluminium
Spodumene: aluminium
Staurolite: aluminium, iron
Stibnite: lead, antimony
Stilbite: aluminium
Sugilite: aluminium
Sulphur
Sunstone: aluminium

T

Tanzanite: aluminium
Tiffany Stone: beryllium
Tiger Eye: asbestos
Topaz: aluminium
Torbernite: *Radioactive*

Tourmaline: aluminium
Tremolite: asbestos
Turquoise: copper and aluminium

U

Ulexite: boron
Unakite: aluminium. (Also zirconium, *Radioactive*.)
Uranophane: *Radioactive*
Uvarovite: aluminium

V

Valentinite: antimony oxide
Vanadinite: vanadium, lead
Variscite: aluminium
Vesuvianite: aluminium
Vivianite: hydrated iron phosphate

W

Wavellite: aluminium
Wulfenite: lead, molybdenum

Z

Zeolite: aluminium
Zircon: zirconium. *Radioactive*
Zoisite: aluminium

Contraindications and cautions

Avoid during full moon: Blue, Cream or Rainbow Moonstone – use Black instead

Bipolar, avoid: Rainbow Mayanite, Red Bushman Quartz, Trigonic Quartz

Catharsis, may induce: Barite, Epidote, Hypersthene, Smoky Spirit Quartz, Tugtupite (replace with Quantum Quattro or Smoky Quartz essence)

Delicate/sensitive people, may overstimulate: Rainbow Moonstone, Red Bushman Quartz, Scolecite, Tanzanite, Tremolite. (Tanzanite may overstimulate psychic abilities as may Rainbow or Blue Moonstone; use black or pink Moonstone instead.)

Depressed: avoid Granite

Dissolves in water: Halite, Hanksite, Selenite

Dizziness, may cause: Preseli Bluestone

Epilepsy: Dumortierite, Geothite, Zircon

Giddiness, remove if causes: Banded Agate

Headache and nausea, if essence causes: Discontinue. Use Smoky Quartz on earth star.

Heart palpitations, avoid: Eilat Stone, Malachite

Hysterical: Avoid Red Bushman Quartz.

Illusion, may induce: Blue or Rainbow Moonstone

Negative energy heightened if used constantly: Epidote, Hypersthene

Pacemakers: Zircon may cause dizziness.

Preseli Bluestone: Do not use in bedroom overnight.

Psychiatric conditions, paranoia or schizophrenia: Do

not use essences unless under the supervision of a qualified crystal healer.

Radioactive: Very dark Smoky Quartz, Uranophane

Tanzanite/Blue Moonstone/Rainbow Moonstone: May create uncontrolled psychic experiences or mental overload or unwanted telepathy.

Toehold in incarnation: Avoid Gabbro with Moonstone, Llanite (Llanoite), Polychrome Jasper. *Chakra:* earth star and soma

Resources

Crystal books by Judy Hall

Volumes in this series

Crystal Prescriptions volume 1: The A-Z guide to over 1,200 symptoms and their healing crystals
Crystal Prescriptions volume 2: The A-Z guide to over 1,250 conditions and their new generation healing crystals
Crystal Prescriptions volume 3: Crystal solutions to electro-magnetic pollution and geopathic stress. An A-Z guide.
Crystal Prescriptions volume 4: The A-Z guide to chakra balancing crystals and kundalini activation stones
Crystal Prescriptions volume 5: Space clearing, Feng Shui and Psychic Protection. An A-Z guide.
Crystal Prescriptions volume 6: Crystals for ancestral clearing, soul retrieval, spirit release and karmic healing. An A-Z guide.

Additional Books

Judy Hall's Crystal Companion (Hamlyn, London, 2018)
The Ultimate Guide to Crystal Grids (Fair Winds Press, USA, January 2018)
The Crystal Bible, volumes 1–3 (Godsfield Press, London, UK. Walking Stick Press, USA)
Earth Blessings: Using Crystals for Personal Energy Clearing, Earth Healing & Environmental Enhancement (Watkins Publishing, 2014)
The Crystal Wisdom Healing Oracle (Watkins Books,

London, 2016)

101 Power Crystals: The Ultimate Guide to Magical Crystals, Gems, and Stones for Healing and Transformation (Fair Winds, USA. Quarto, London)

Crystals and Sacred Sites: Use Crystals to Access the Power of Sacred Landscapes for Personal and Planetary Transformation (Fair Winds, USA, 2012)

Good Vibrations: Psychic Protection, Energy Enhancement and Space Clearing (Flying Horse Publications, Bournemouth)

Further Reading

If you wish to create essences for sale or to understand the underlying principles of essence creation in depth, you can do no better than consult Sue Lilly, *The Essence Practitioner*, Singing Dragon, London, 2015.

Baines, Tracey, *It's not about the food: Battling through your child's eating disorder* (The Meggie Press, 2017)

Cunningham, Donna, MSW, and Andrew Ramer, *Spiritual Dimensions of Healing Addictions* and *Further Dimensions of Healing Addictions* (Cassandra Press, 1988 and 1989)

Henry Cornelius Agrippa of Nettesheim, *Three Books of Occult Philosophy* (Llewellyn, St Paul, MN, 2004 version)

Kunz, George Frederick, *The Curious Lore of Precious Stones* (Dover, New York, 1971 reprint)

If you wish to discover the ancient healing powers of crystals, Pliny, *Natural History Books 16–17*, Loeb Classical

Library, translated by D.E. Eichholz (Harvard University Press, Cambridge, 1962), also covers the stones in the much referenced but difficult to obtain *Theophrastus on Stones*, translated by Earle R. Caley and John C. Richards (Columbus: Ohio State University, 1956).

Essence suppliers

Petaltone Essences: www.petaltone.co.uk, www.petaltoneusa.com, www.petaltone-jp.com

The Crystal Balance Company: www.crystalbalance.co.uk

Crystal suppliers

John van Rees, Exquisite Crystals: www.exquisite-crystals.com

Judy Hall via http://www.astrologywise.co.uk/store---crystals-jewelry-downloads.html

Spiritual Planet: www.spiritualplanet.co.uk – who also supply essences.

The planetary hours

Calculator: http://www.astrology.com.tr/planetary-hours.asp and http://www.lunarium.co.uk/planets/hours.jsp and see

http://www.renaissanceastrology.com/planetaryhoursarticle.html and http://chronosxp.sourceforge.net/en/hours.html

Fixed stars

Brady's Book of Fixed Stars, Red Wheel/Weiser; New edition 1 October 1999

http://www.renaissanceastrology.com/hermesfixedstars.html gives the English translation of the annoyingly untranslated Latin names of the gems associated with fifteen of the fixed stars found in Appendix G of Joan Evans, *Magical Jewels of the Middles Ages and the Renaissance Particularly in England*, Dover Publications, New York, undated.

Endnotes

1. Introduction to *The Essence Practitioner*, Sue Lilly (Singing Dragon, London, 2015)
2. Pliny the Elder, *Natural History, Books XIV, XII:85 etc.*
3. Pliny, *Book XXXVII*, LIV 143
4. Pliny, *Book XXXVI*
5. *Mystical and Mythological Explanatory Works of Assyrian and Babylonian Scholars* (Clarendon Press, Oxford, 1986)
6. Combined from Kunz, *Curious Lore of Precious Stones.*
7. See *Crystal Prescriptions volume 3* for full reference and research findings.
8. See *Crystal Prescriptions volume 5* and *The Ultimate Guide to Crystal Grids* for grid patterns.

BOOKS

O-BOOKS

SPIRITUALITY

O is a symbol of the world, of oneness and unity; this eye represents knowledge and insight. We publish titles on general spirituality and living a spiritual life. We aim to inform and help you on your own journey in this life. If you have enjoyed this book, why not tell other readers by posting a review on your preferred book site?

Recent bestsellers from O-Books are:

Heart of Tantric Sex
Diana Richardson
Revealing Eastern secrets of deep love and intimacy to
Western couples.
Paperback: 978-1-90381-637-0 ebook: 978-1-84694-637-0

Crystal Prescriptions
The A-Z guide to over 1,200 symptoms and their healing
crystals
Judy Hall
The first in the popular series of eight books, this handy
little guide is packed as tight as a pill-bottle with crystal
remedies for ailments.
Paperback: 978-1-90504-740-6 ebook: 978-1-84694-629-5

Take Me To Truth
Undoing the Ego
Nouk Sanchez, Tomas Vieira
The best-selling step-by-step book on shedding the Ego,
using the teachings of *A Course In Miracles*.
Paperback: 978-1-84694-050-7 ebook: 978-1-84694-654-7

The 7 Myths about Love...Actually!
The journey from your HEAD to the HEART of your SOUL
Mike George
Smashes all the myths about LOVE.
Paperback: 978-1-84694-288-4 ebook: 978-1-84694-682-0

The Holy Spirit's Interpretation of the New Testament
A Course in Understanding and Acceptance
Regina Dawn Akers
Following on from the strength of *A Course In Miracles*,
NTI teaches us how to experience the love and oneness
of God.
Paperback: 978-1-84694-085-9 ebook: 978-1-78099-083-5

The Message of A Course In Miracles
A translation of the text in plain language
Elizabeth A. Cronkhite
A translation of *A Course in Miracles* into plain, everyday
language for anyone seeking inner peace. The
companion volume, *Practicing A Course In Miracles*,
offers practical lessons and mentoring.
Paperback: 978-1-84694-319-5 ebook: 978-1-84694-642-4

Thinker's Guide to God
Peter Vardy
An introduction to key issues in the philosophy of
religion.
Paperback: 978-1-90381-622-6

Your Simple Path
Find happiness in every step
Ian Tucker
A guide to helping us reconnect with what is really
important in our lives.
Paperback: 978-1-78279-349-6 ebook: 978-1-78279-348-9

The Ecology of the Soul
A Manual of Peace, Power and Personal Growth for Real
People in the Real World
Aidan Walker
Balance your own inner Ecology of the Soul to regain
your natural state of peace, power and wellbeing.
Paperback: 978-1-78279-850-7 ebook: 978-1-78279-849-1

Not I, Not other than I
The Life and Teachings of Russel Williams
Steve Taylor, Russel Williams
The miraculous life and inspiring teachings of one of the
World's greatest living Sages.
Paperback: 978-1-78279-729-6 ebook: 978-1-78279-728-9

On the Other Side of Love
A Woman's Unconventional Journey Towards Wisdom
Muriel Maufroy
When life has lost all meaning, what do you do?
Paperback: 978-1-78535-281-2 ebook: 978-1-78535-282-9

Practicing A Course In Miracles
A Translation of the Workbook in Plain Language and
With Mentoring Notes
Elizabeth A. Cronkhite
The practical second and third volumes of The Plain-
Language *A Course In Miracles*.
Paperback: 978-1-84694-403-1 ebook: 978-1-78099-072-9

Quantum Bliss
The Quantum Mechanics of Happiness, Abundance, and
Health
George S. Mentz
Quantum Bliss is the breakthrough summary of success
and spirituality secrets that customers have been
waiting for.
Paperback: 978-1-78535-203-4 ebook: 978-1-78535-204-1

The Upside Down Mountain
Mags MacKean
A must-read for anyone weary of chasing success and
happiness – one woman's inspirational journey
swapping the uphill slog for the downhill slope.
Paperback: 978-1-78535-171-6 ebook: 978-1-78535-172-3

Your Personal Tuning Fork
The Endocrine System
Deborah Bates
Discover your body's health secret, the endocrine
system, and 'twang' your way to sustainable health!
Paperback: 978-1-84694-503-8 ebook: 978-1-78099-697-4

Readers of ebooks can buy or view any of these bestsellers by clicking on the live link in the title. Most titles are published in paperback and as an ebook. Paperbacks are available in traditional bookshops. Both print and ebook formats are available online.

Find more titles and sign up to our readers' newsletter at http://www.johnhuntpublishing.com/mind-body-spirit

Follow us on Facebook at
https://www.facebook.com/OBooks/